TIMEBOMB

TIMEBOMB

A WAR on HUMAN GENETICS!

A Genocide of DEADLY Processed Foods!

A National Health Epidemic More Pervasive Than Anyone Imagined!

Don't Be Its Next VICTIM!

JOE HORN
& ALLIE ANDERSON

Defender

Crane, MO

TIMEBOMB

Joe Horn & Allie Anderson

With contributors: Dr. Matthew Sams, DC, FIACA, Dr. Joshua Vance, DC, MTAA, Dr. Ralph A. Umbriaco, DC, MsTOM, CNHP

Defender Crane, MO 65633 ©2018. All rights reserved.

Published 2018. Printed in the United States of America.

ISBN: 9781948014014

A CIP catalog record of this book is available from the Library of Congress.

Cover illustration and design by Jeffrey Mardis.

All Scripture quotations from the King James Version; in cases of academic comparison, those instances are noted.

DEDICATION

This book is dedicated to my beautiful wife Katherine, who has carried me through so much; to my amazing children; and to the countless friends and family members who have lifted me up through prayer.

   —Joe Horn

This book is dedicated to my children, John and Kat: May you always follow the Lord and live out every wonderful thing He has for you. I want to thank my family for all their love and support, and most of all, God, for all He has brought me through, and the wonderful new people He has brought into my life.

   —Allie Anderson

contents

A Note to the Reader:

The phrase "CAM (Complementary and Alternative Medicine) Therapy" is a blanket phrase used to address any type of medical practice that is found outside the realm of traditional, modern, American medical practice. This can include acupuncture, osteopathic or chiropractic practices, holistic medicine, homeopathic medicine, naturopathic practices, massage therapy, physical therapy, and more. In the part of this book contributed by Dr. Matthew Sams, DC, FIACA, variations between available types of CAM practices are outlined and more thoroughly explained to the reader, but for practical purposes, throughout the main body of this book, I will be using the phrase "holistic" to refer to any and all natural or alternative medicine. In no way am I suggesting that readers limit themselves to any one alternative medical practitioner by means of title, as many qualified and knowledgeable individuals, for a variety of reasons, may operate under different labels included under the blanket phrase of CAM Therapy.

1

My Story

I didn't know where to turn. Although I had been sick off and on for years, I had never been in *this dire* a situation. This time, I was *really* in trouble. The infection inside me was raging, more painful than ever, and had hit an all new level of toxic. I was on my third—and final—week of antibiotics. My doctor had previously told me that if the infection could not be controlled by the antibiotics, there was a good chance that it could turn septic inside my intestines and possibly even rupture, resulting in a frantic, life-or-death trip to the ER along with an emergency surgery with whatever doctor happened to be on duty at the time. I was petrified of landing in such a scenario, yet despite taking preventative measures, I felt as if such a crisis was unavoidable. My general practitioner could prescribe more antibiotics for me, but since the ones I had already been taking for the past two weeks were making no difference this time around, I knew that simply was not a solution. I was aware, based on my previous experiences and advice from the many doctors I had seen over the past decade, that the time for surgery had come. I couldn't put it off any longer. With the situation escalating to the point that my doctors had always predicted it would, I phoned my specialist's office, talking to the nurse and telling her that the symptoms were rapidly approaching the inevitable point the doctor had warned me about.

What happened next stunned me. I learned that my specialist's software had purged my name and information from his client base. Since it had been more than a year since my last appointment, I would now have to be treated like a new patient. The nurse assured me that the staff remembered my situation well, but, due to recent changes within the medical industry, there were policies to be followed and unavoidable formalities. Intake for new a patient would take sixty to ninety days. I pleaded with the nurse to recheck the doctor's calendar for a new patient appointment sooner, reminding her I had been warned that if the situation in my colon ever turned septic or ruptured, I risked ending up in the ER—not only in agonizing pain, but facing a potentially infectious, possibly fatal, surgery. Since the antibiotics were not able to curb any of the pain I was in and my relentless symptoms refused to subside on any level, I knew I was out of time. This turn of events, however, was like having the rug pulled out from under me. I had been told previously that the illness had to "play itself out" in order for my medical insurance to cover the surgery. Because of this, the doctor wouldn't perform surgery before it was unavoidable, forcing me to wait until the illness had advanced, thus warranting medical insurance coverage. It had been a strange game of "hurry up and wait."

The scenario unfolding around me seemed like a bad dream I hoped to wake up from at any moment. I had never expected to find myself without medical care. I had anticipated calling the specialist, telling him that the symptoms had finally hit their worst and letting him know it was time to act. I had imagined that he would respond by getting me into his office quickly and scheduling a quick surgery.

Since this wasn't the way it played out with my doctor, I called several other physicians to see if they could get me in sooner, and each gave the same answer: "We can do a new patient intake and see you within thirty to ninety days, and if the doctor feels you are a candidate for surgery, we can certainly schedule that for you."

I was out of options, completely vulnerable, and afraid. I felt like I was carrying a timebomb, and my plan for defusing it had fallen apart. I could try my primary care doctor again; I was certain she would agree to prescribe more antibiotics, but her participation wouldn't likely help me much. Since the antibiotics were no longer bringing about any relief whatsoever for my symptoms, it was obvious they weren't curing the infection. And the infection was the timebomb that doctors had been warning me about all along. For years, when I had asked questions about the impending arrival of this day, they had given generic instructions such as, "If it gets dangerous, you'll know. It'll be such unbelievable pain, with no relief whatsoever. And if you get to that point, *get to ER right away, because it can be dangerous.* Don't waste any time. Drop what you're doing and get to a hospital immediately."

The physical pain and anxiety were unbearable. I was terrified. For years, I had trusted my many doctors' wisdom. I had followed their advice and paid attention to the symptoms they told me to watch for. Now that the symptoms were here, there seemed to be no help for me. I made myself breathe in and out…in and out…pacing myself through each moment…trying to hold the anxiety at bay until some idea would surface as to where I could turn for help. I was pulling into a parking spot at work, praying for a miracle, when my phone went off announcing the arrival of a text message. It was from my dear friend, Caspar McCloud. He was aware of my health issues, and I had texted him earlier the same morning asking for prayer.

I looked down at the text message that had just beeped my phone:

Expect healing to overtake you in the almighty name of Jesus.

The very moment my eyes finished reading the text, falling on the words "name of Jesus," the phone rang. I answered it, the last fragments of hope hanging at the end of my voice by a thread.

"Is Joe Horn available?" came the female voice on the other end of the line.

"This is he," I answered. The caller explained that she was getting in touch with me on behalf of one of the surgeons in the area, whom I later found out was one of the most skilled in this region. The call was in response to a plea for help a friend of mine within the medical field had put out on my behalf. My eyes fought the urge to flood with tears that had been toying at their edges all morning long. I'm not sure I heard every word the caller said in the following moments, but I did hear this: "Are you available tomorrow morning at 9 AM for an appointment?"

At that moment, the dam broke, and the tears flowed. After nearly fifteen years of suffering from a debilitating chronic illness that had stolen my quality of life, plagued my mind on sleepless nights, and danced at the edges of my peripheral vision as the possible harbinger of life-threatening disaster, I was about to find healing.

But, despite an efficient and skilled surgeon and a predictably adequate recovery process, the healing did not come the way I expected, nor did a sudden, spiritual lightning bolt flash from the sky and heal me immediately. The healing was not even a *direct* result of the surgery I finally underwent. Rather, the *real* healing has been through the journey that began *after* my surgery. It has been a slow path that has required diligence and true seeking, one breadcrumb at a time. The path to healing I've found is one I never would have suspected, and it is definitely the road less traveled, a road that is straight and narrow…

—

I grew up as a pretty healthy kid, in a home with both parents, and Mom stayed home and packed our school lunches and made dinner each night. As a teenager, my life got busy, and I graduated high school early to begin working. By the time I was 20, I was working full time during the week (forty-plus hours from Monday to Friday) selling convenience food and working a second part-time job on the weekends (ten-to twelve-hour shifts on Saturdays and Sundays). In addition to those two activities, I played my guitar in youth group bands every chance I got. I suppose, looking back, that the first indicator I would've had that I was dealing with inflammation would have been the tendinitis that occasionally interfered with my guitar playing during these years, but at the time, I disregarded it, assuming it was as normal as the tendinitis I had heard other, older guitar players complain about.

By the time I was 24, I was a recreational director at a huge camp and conference facility. I was a rec-tech-certified high-ropes course and zipline instructor facilitator and a certified American Red Cross lifeguard instructor trainer. I held a diploma from the Oregon State Sanitary Services Department for completing water quality and pool management training. I managed all recreational facilities and staff and oversaw maintenance on the various recreational equipment. I was required to physically be able to do each duty that fell under these parameters, including the distance swimming required for lifeguards, maneuvering all the elements in the high and low ropes courses, conducting emergency takedowns from the sixty-foot-high, rope-course line (a maneuver that involved safely removing an individual from a ropes course, should the need arise), and loading and unloading all equipment such as paddleboats and bicycles. At a height of 6 feet, 2 inches, and weighing 179 pounds, during that time in my life, I was the most physically fit I've ever been.

My beautiful newlywed wife, Katherine, worked alongside me. We lived on site and were provided with the benefit of being able to eat in the camp cafeteria any time a meal was provided for the group of campers. We had it made. Yet, despite my appearance of health, I was already wrestling with physical issues behind the scenes. At times, the symptoms were so subtle or so sporadic that I often attributed them to aging, being tired, or just eating something that didn't agree with me. The only real, constant two symptoms I recall experiencing this early on were feeling that no matter how much I slept, I never felt rested, and a constant alternation between having diarrhea and constipation. It was easy to attribute problems like those to my demanding job that kept me running all day long for many months out of the year. Whenever I mentioned it, people who were older than me would laugh and say, "Yeah, and it doesn't get any better the older you get!"

When I got my first urinary tract infection (UTI) during those days, my doctor regarded it as strange, since it's a pretty unusual condition for a man. He put me on antibiotics, and I went about my business for about six months—until I got a second UTI. Soon, this became a repetitive predicament, so my doctor decided to do some further checking. After running a cytoscopy, or bladder scope, I was told that I had chronic bacterial prostatitis and that this was the reason I was now averaging two bladder infections a year. I continued to intermittently be put on antibiotics until finally my doctor performed an intravenous pyelogram (a procedure in which an iodine-based contrast dye is injected and then equipment is used to view the kidneys). This ruled out bladder cancer and all other logical culprits. As a last resort, my doctor prescribed a ninety-day round of antibiotics to kill any lingering infection.

About eight months later, I woke up in the middle of the night feeling like I had a bad case of the flu, except that something wasn't quite the same as a regular viral bug. I felt as though I was running a high temperature and my body ached and trembled all over. I was incredibly nauseous. Light hurt my eyes. I could hardly move, and it was all I could do to get to the car so my wife could drive me to the hospital. I was too weak to get out of the car; she had to get a wheelchair and help me seat myself in it so that she could get me into the emergency room. After a series of lab tests were run, the doctor informed me that I had E. coli. Katherine and I immediately began to review what foods I had eaten until the doctor said that I had the kind of E. coli the body generates when the digestive track isn't operating properly. He couldn't fully explain the cause, but because of the chronic constipation I was suffering, he speculated that something had "backed up," become infected, and generated this bacteria within my intestine.

I was given another round of antibiotics and had a colonoscopy, which showed nothing.

During all of this, Katherine and I decided we wanted a child. We tried repeatedly for her to become pregnant, and we became one of those couples who lived on the emotional merry-go-round of getting our hopes up each month, only to have them dashed again when we realized Katherine hadn't conceived. For a while, we thought this was normal. After all, who gets pregnant the first month or two? But after some time, we decided to have some tests run to determine the underlying problem. My wife checked out just fine. I, on the other hand, showed a sperm count of 1000. My doctor informed me that anything lower than 20 to 40 million was considered low. This put me at such a minuscule amount, he told me, that it was doubtful my wife could *ever* become pregnant. After this devastating blow, we knew we had three options: artificial insemination, in vitro fertilization, or adoption. We prayed about it, weighing economical, spiritual, and relational pros and cons of each option, and finally decided that adoption was the best route for us. My wife, filled with new zeal and hope, began to pursue this option, only to see every open door slam shut. At this time, we were earnestly seeking God's will, and knew that He had the best plan in mind, but it was discouraging to constantly meet a dead end. (Praise God—we've now been blessed with four beautiful children, but that's another story.)

Because of the infertility issues we were facing, I followed one doctor's recommendation to have a varicocele procedure done, which would, I was told, address the issue of low sperm count (caused by inflammation in my testicles, which they speculated could be overheating and killing my sperm). By now, I was still experiencing tendon inflammation on mild levels in addition to the ever-mounting fatigue and alternating constipation and diarrhea. On top of these symptoms, I also began to have adult acne that manifest in the form of boils all over my head and scalp. I began to experience intermittent surges of anxiety, along with an underlying nervous tension that seemed to accompany me all my waking hours. It felt like I was racing through life, running on adrenaline instead of the natural energy accumulated during sleep. I asked my doctors about these things, and any tests they ran were always inconclusive.

Throughout all of this, not one doctor ever mentioned the importance of diet.

The doctor who performed my varicocele predicted that within a year my sperm count would show improvement, which turned out to be true. Shortly after that, Katherine became pregnant with our first child. Over the course of my treatment with that doctor, he also recommended that I take saw palmetto, which I did for about two years. Having no understanding of its connection to my actual problems, one day when I ran out of the supplement, I simply didn't buy any more.

It seemed for a while that my health might have been improving after the varicocele. After all, my sperm count had risen and, as I mentioned, my wife had become pregnant. But I still had the fatigue, nervous energy, surges of anxiety, acne, and gut pains that contributed to the alternating constipation and diarrhea. Life would get easier for a while and the pain in my guts would subside, only to escalate again, while the diarrhea and constipation would worsen. This cycle continued for about five years. During this time, I also struggled with intermittent chest pains that would come on so suddenly and painfully that I eventually had a doctor check my heart. He ran a series of tests and finally diagnosed me with pleurisy, which he said was caused by inflammation on the lining of my lung. I learned how to identify and breathe through the episodes, and life went on.

By the time I was 30, I had settled into a more sedentary job, which mostly required me to sit behind a computer. My complexion had become pasty, and I weighed nearly 260 pounds. The acne boils on my head were so profound that they were visible through my hair. The pain in my gut had slowly increased, and chronic constipation had become a way of life. I was also burning the candle at both ends, working too many hours and dealing with a lot of stress at work. Because of all I was juggling, I wasn't keeping regularly structured work, sleeping, or eating times. I would work a long day, come home and grab a Hot Pocket, go back to work for several more hours, come back home, binge-eat Froot Loops at midnight, go to bed at 2 AM, wake up at 7 AM, and do the whole thing again. I knew I couldn't keep this pace forever, but I had seen many other people in ministry do this very thing. I assumed burning myself out in this way was the same as giving my all to God.

By 2009, because of all the stress I was carrying at the time, my anxiety had slowly reached a new level. The constant nervous energy of adrenaline that had previously lingered beneath the surface had escalated to a continuous, buzzing undercurrent. One night, in an episode very similar to the one the night I had been diagnosed with E. coli those years earlier, I woke up in the wee hours with a terrible pain in my gut, worse than I had ever felt. Again, I thought I was dying. This pain was even more intense than I had endured the previous night nearly five years earlier. Katherine took me to the hospital, where I underwent myriad tests, including a second colonoscopy and a CT scan. This time, however, the tests were not inconclusive. The diagnosis was diverticulitis, caused by diverticulosis, a condition that causes small, pouch-type polyps to appear inside the wall of the large intestine. Over time, they can become infected, causing the diverticulitis. Somehow, within the five years since my last colonoscopy, my colon had gone from looking perfectly clean to being filled with nodes. I had known for a while that something wasn't right in my intestinal tract, but receiving this news really scared me.

I had never thought of myself as a person who might actually have a disease. Not only was the doctor now telling me that I did *indeed* have a disease, but that it was incurable, and I would likely have it for the rest of my life. His reassurances were statements such as "This is a pretty common disease" and "It can be hereditary, genetic even. Lots of people have it and manage it on a daily basis."

One thing about this bothered me a lot. In fact, looking back, it really stuck with me. The doctor who performed the colonoscopy told me, "You just had your first infection. By the time you have your third infection, you'll be a candidate for surgery." When I asked him what he meant, he told me they might eventually need to remove the infected part of my colon. I remember being stunned at the idea that he could be so casual about possibly cutting out part of my body. His answer to my concern was simple: "Just don't worry about right now." I remember asking him if there was anything I could do to prevent this possible future complication. He responded that it was hereditary, and there wasn't anything that could be done. He added that it never hurts to take fiber and lose some weight.

He also said if it became infected, it could be dangerous. I remember asking how to tell if it was infected or dangerous.

"Oh, you'll know!" he said. "You'll know if you get infected, because it's *extremely* painful." And, I remember him adding, "If you ever think you have an infection, get the problem addressed right away. If it becomes septic it can be deadly."

On that, I obtained my prescription for another round of antibiotics and left the hospital feeling somewhat lost. I had never been told that I had an incurable disease. Stopping on my way home at a big-box grocery store, I filled my prescription for antibiotics and bought an inexpensive fiber (which I later learned was made at such low-quality standards that it held nearly no nutritional benefit), determined to try to prioritize my health better than I had previously. I took the antibiotics as directed by my doctor. By this time, every bowel movement was extremely painful, so that made remembering to take my fiber pretty easy. Over the next few years, my health fluctuated between "really bad" and "less bad." When I went through times when I felt a little bit better, I would "slip" and forget to take my fiber (which I later learned probably saved me from lazy bowel disorder, a condition caused by living on laxatives wherein your gut is being trained to stop contracting in an effort to make bowel movement happen at all, because of the addictive, synthetic, artificially sweetened, and orange-colored fiber I was using at the time). On the other hand, working one's gut so hard all the time has side effects. Because the gut is the second brain (to be discussed later in this book), common side effects of diverticulitis include depression or anxiety. My anxiety continued to be an issue, and at times I even had doctors offer me antidepressants. Not wanting to go that route, I continued to bolster my resolve to fight for my health.

I had always loved martial arts, and I knew exercise was healthy, so I decided to start working out by practicing martial arts. Twice a week, I went to an especially strenuous class that involved high-level cardio workouts for an hour at a time. I also did sparring exercises, went running several times a week, and went through training programs like some that the UFC (Ultimate Fighting Championship) fighters do. I turned my basement into a gym, working heavy bags and punching bags at home in between class days. I lost fifty pounds in three months, bringing my weight down to 201 pounds. As hard as I tried, I never could crack that two-hundred-pound mark, and I never lost the actual "belly fat." On top of this, I continued to feel sick, fatigued, and plagued by the same symptoms I had been dealing with now for years. Any additional doctors I saw parroted the same advice or diagnosis I had already been given.

I couldn't understand why, despite my efforts, I wasn't getting any better. I was even watching what I was eating. I wasn't on any official diet to speak of, but I was avoiding breads and trying to stay away from sugar. I watched many episodes of *The Biggest Loser* during that chapter of my life, and generally followed the dietary guidelines taught to the competitors on that show. If they were told to eat more fruit, I remembered that the next time I went grocery shopping. If they were told that kale was a good idea, I added it to my next salad. I was counting my blessings, praying each day, and doing devotions along with my Bible reading. Despite the weight loss and all the other changes I was making for the better, I continued to feel more fatigued, sicker, and more irregular than ever. The anxiety and adult acne were also worse than they had ever been. Finally, in 2012, I became so sick I couldn't keep up with the workouts anymore. By this time, my wife and I had two daughters, and my wife was pregnant with our third. Sadly, this pregnancy ended in miscarriage, and the devastation I faced zapped any fight I had left to continue this intense routine. I stopped going to karate, and the workouts ceased. I slowly gained back the weight. (I later realized that doing these strenuous exercises was one of the worst things I could do, considering the condition of my health, because of the demand it placed on my already-depleted adrenals.)

Over the years, I had seen multiple other doctors and received other diagnoses similar to diverticulosis and diverticulitis, such as irritable bowel syndrome, inflammatory bowel disease, nervous bowel disease, spastic colon, and nervous colon. Although I was initially willing to try all the prescriptions I was given, I never felt any relief and eventually stopped taking the medication. I have had hormone testing, blood testing, various panels showing blood levels on the many types of criteria specialists deemed necessary, and many other tests by well-meaning doctors who were trying to get to the root of my problem. Neither antibiotics nor anti-inflammatories gave me any relief. Each time a new round of tests was run, or I was referred to another doctor, I went through a waiting period during which I held a tepid hope that the next doctor would be the one to have an answer that could help me. Each test I waited for was another period of hours, days, or sometimes weeks of suspense. Sometimes we prayed the doctors would not find anything; other times, we prayed they would find *something*. And, over the years, I was continually offered anti-anxiety meds, which I always declined.

I can't fully explain why I didn't want to take these medicines. Somehow, deep down, I knew that what I was dealing with was springing from a deeper cause. I had watched friends go on these meds, and while some seemed to experience relief from their anxiety, many felt an overall "sleepiness" or "numbness." For many people I had seen, it didn't appear to be possible to isolate the anxiety and adjust that without changing other aspects of their reactive personality as well. I was glad for those I knew who benefited from using these medications, but something in my soul told me that wasn't the solution I was looking for. For me, it was somehow a door I never felt comfortable to open. Besides, I was aware that the anxiety stemmed from the fact that I knew something was wrong with me that the doctors were not finding. Combining this unspoken knowledge with the doctors' statements that what little they *were* able to diagnose was simply "hereditary and incurable" caused a foreboding sense that when they finally did find an underlying diagnosis, I would just have to shrug and accept that as well.

Yet, throughout all of this, no one ever suggested I look at diet as a solution.

By 2014, the inflammation throughout my stomach region was so pronounced that my midsection changed sizes almost daily. Pants that fit me one day would not zip up the next. One day, my stomach looked bloated, and the next day, I appeared thinner. This time, when the diverticulitis infection struck for the second time in all its fury— with indescribable pain in my gut, high fevers, irregularity (even more so than usual), and intense inflammation—I recognized the symptoms and went to a doctor right away. Another round of antibiotics. The emergency room staffers told me that if I didn't see improvement after taking the course of the antibiotics, I should follow up with my regular gastroenterologist. Because the antibiotics took me from "horrible" status back up to my usual "really painful" status, I didn't do that follow-up. Little did I know that this deviation in judgment would cause my patient status to become inactive within that specialist's computer software, thus I would be purged as a patient, as mentioned earlier.

Over the previous several years, I had developed a friendship with my chiropractor, Dr. Joshua Vance. One day, during an appointment when he was adjusting my back, the subject of my intestinal pain came up. Joshua, who not only is a chiropractor, but also a certified CBP, MTAA who is working toward his DABCI, encouraged me to consider pursuing a natural route of treatment. It was hard to imagine that he might know how to treat my gut in the condition it was in, with all its complicated history. I had no doubt that Joshua knew what he was talking about, but I hesitated at the idea that natural methods could still help *me*. I could easily see how a person sticking to an all-natural diet and turning to holistic and herbal remedies from a young age would be able to maintain consistent health using only natural means. But for a person with my medical history—considering all the processed foods I had eaten, the many rounds of antibiotics my stomach had endured, the escalated inflammation, damage from diverticulosis and outbreaks of diverticulitis, colonoscopies, varicocele, and other procedures that I had been through—it seemed inconceivable that simply turning to a natural remedy could *reverse* the damage that had taken place over all those years. Besides, with "modern medical wonders" as evolved as they are, surely these medical treatments would have been as effective as anything available in the natural world, with the added benefit of advanced science? Moreover, the fact that I was dealing with a chronic condition meant I was almost guaranteed it would return. I was having a hard time believing natural methods could get ahead of my escalating health problems, considering my history of chronic infection.

In early 2016, my problems had intensified to the point that they affected every aspect of my life. My energy was at an all-time low. I couldn't play with my children, and enduring even a regular day at work had become a challenge. We changed our family activities to accommodate my short-termed stamina. My wife became used to taking our children to activities without me, knowing that my core responsibilities were all I could handle anymore. My gut pain alternated constantly between dull, aching pains that moved from side to side across my abdomen to sharp, stabbing pains that bounced around sporadically. The fatigue was so bad that I drank coffee all day long just to stay awake. No matter how early I went to bed, I never got enough sleep. I eliminated all extra "commitments" to conserve energy for responsibilities that were nonnegotiable. And when diverticulitis hit again in 2016, harder than ever, I remembered the words of that doctor so many years ago who had put such an omen over infection number *three*.

In the same style as the previous two episodes, this one hit at 2 o'clock in the morning. As before, my amazing wife Katherine took me to the hospital. Lab work was run, blood was drawn, CT scans were performed, and I was given another round of antibiotics. This time, however, was different. I took the antibiotics as instructed, but the pain was relentless. Even as I finished the medications, I felt no relief. The agony, worse than any outbreak up to now, didn't subside even slightly under the medication. I knew this was what I had been warned about: The doctor told me that when it was truly dangerous, it would be so painful I would have no doubt about it and there would be no relief. He had *also* warned me that when it got to that point, I should not go untreated. I had been cautioned that the infection could become resistant to the antibiotics and that it could escalate within a person's body until it becomes septic, allowing opportunity for the affected internal organ to potentially burst, creating a possibly fatal emergency. I called the specialist I had seen in 2009, only to find out that, because it had been more than a year since my last appointment with him, I had been purged as a patient. My primary care doctor was able to offer more antibiotics and a referral to a specialist, but that didn't address the ticking timebomb now raging in my abdomen. After all these years of being warned, I found myself in the very situation I had most feared all along. I just *knew* I was infected with another round of diverticulitis, but this time, my body had not responded to the antibiotics, the specialist had purged me from his patient list, and the best my primary care physician could do was give me more of the same medicine that already wasn't working. My emergency backup plan had become to hope my intestines didn't become septic or rupture before I could get into surgery.

Expect healing to overtake you in the almighty name of Jesus.

The phone rang, and it was the nurse from a local surgeon's office—the one who had responded to Joshua Vance's plea for help on my behalf. Joshua didn't want to see me have surgery, and he had made that clear. But, he also understood that I had been told I would eventually need surgery and that I was convinced the time had arrived. I was offered an appointment the next morning at 9 o'clock—a miracle all by itself—and I went. After examining me, the surgeon confirmed that I did indeed need sixteen inches of my colon removed.

I was thrilled to have the surgery scheduled. After fifteen years of battling an illness that had made me suffer constantly, I knew I was about to gain a new lease on life. This newfound hope of healing kept me optimistic during these days.

Katherine, during this time, was pregnant with (and later delivered) our fourth child. During her third and fourth pregnancies, she had become increasingly interested in natural forms of medication and treatment and chose to use a midwife instead of a traditional hospital for her obstetric care and deliveries. Throughout this journey, her awareness of natural remedies began to increase. Before my surgery, she went with me to one of my appointments to see the surgeon and asked him if probiotics could possibly alleviate any of my symptoms or improve my condition. He told her that taking them probably wouldn't hurt anything, but that there was "no science to back the idea that they would help." The doctor said it would be at least three months before I was well enough to perform my usual duties at work and home, but I just *knew* I would beat that deadline. After all, I was getting a new lease on life. I couldn't wait.

The procedure was scheduled within days and went smoothly—exactly the way the surgeon had said it would. He had warned that my recovery would be slow—and it stood to reason, since my health had been so bad before the surgery. He was telling me the truth. This was one of the most painful, slowest recoveries I could've ever imagined. I had nausea unlike during any flu I've ever had. It was kind of like motion sickness, as if the room were constantly moving. I would close my eyes to sleep, but my sleep was interrupted by strange, nervous dreams. These dreams were often repetitive and continued throughout the night in sudden, nonsensical flashes. Sometimes, in these dreams, I saw myself floating over the ocean or spinning in circles under the stars, then I would awake to a whole new wave of indescribable nausea. The closest thing I can compare it to would be the repetitive, nerve-wracking, nonsensical dreams people have when they are running an extremely high temperature.

For months, my gut remained in excruciating pain. The constipation was worse than I had ever experienced, and bowel movements were unbearable. The nausea made it impossible to keep anything down, which also slowed my recovery. I spent those first three months remembering when I was young, before this illness had stuck my life. During that time, I constantly prayed under my breath, *Lord Jesus,* please *let this chapter of my life be over.* Please *let this chapter end. I just want to get back to being well. Please, Lord Jesus, please, take me back to a normal life.*

During this journey, Katherine began to search for ways she could help me with the nausea. I lost a lot of weight during that time and had that pale, gaunt look of being sick and underweight. My inability to keep food down was becoming an increasing concern, and she wanted to find foods my body could absorb. Katherine had always been one to cook meals at home, but during this time, she began to increasingly eliminate processed foods from the grocery list. She bought a pressure cooker and began to make stew-type meals in bone broth, as well as other recipes she found online that looked like they might help me. She also began to use the word "natural" more often. One day, she brought some essential oils into the living room where I was lying on the couch. I remember her saying that the peppermint oil should help.

"I'm too sick; take it out of here. I can't handle the smell," I remember saying.

"Just try it, honey," she said. "I've been reading about it online, I really think it will help you."

I remember manufacturing enough humor to tell her that I was too sick to try her "snake oil," and asking her to put the lid on it before the smell made me even more nauseous. She consented and left the room.

Over the next couple of days, she became more insistent until I finally agreed to try the peppermint oil. At first, I couldn't tell how my body would respond. But after a couple of minutes, the nausea subsided slightly. Over the following days, I came to a point that I couldn't stand to be away from that oil. I formed the habit of taking the lid off and holding the entire bottle beneath my nose at the first sign of nausea. Soon, I started noticing a change: I was beginning to rely on the reprieve it offered from the nausea.

Throughout this period, Joshua Vance continued to encourage me to explore the natural route toward healing. Several other friends were beginning to use the phrase "natural healing" as well. It was as if the phrase was suddenly emerging as a common theme in many different areas of my life. Even those who texted me to let me know they were praying for me would encourage me to look into "natural healing" without any prompting at all on my part. Because of my experience with the oil, I was more open-minded to natural alternatives than I had been previously, but I was still waiting for that moment when I would be fully recovered from the surgery and *back* to being healthy before I felt I could really explore the option. It was as though I expected to be given a clean slate after the recovery process, and *from there* I planned to consider adapting myself to a more natural lifestyle. I couldn't seem to get my head to let go of the idea that to go forward in a natural way, I would have to be "cleared" by the medical world first.

In the meantime, my continued pain after surgery made me concerned that there had been a complication with my recovery, or that they might not have removed all the diverticulosis. I started thinking about how long the large intestine was and began worrying that the sixteen inches they had taken might not have removed the core issue. I was haunted by a lingering fear that a more nefarious condition might be lurking further in the remaining segment of my colon, something perhaps the doctors had missed. I repeatedly went back to my surgeon to make sure that I was doing as expected. The pain lingered so drastically that I wondered if I had somehow ripped one of the areas that had been reattached during the surgery. The doctor's answer to this concern was strangely similar to answers I had heard for other questions I had asked in the past: "It's highly unlikely that you've torn anything in there. If you do that, you'll know. It will be so painful you'll be in ER before you know it." And with those generic instructions, I was sent on my way. I continued to plod through my "recovery," both taking solace in and having dread for the fact that the pain was nearly identical to what I had experienced before the surgery. I lived on the faith that if I had torn something or there was a further complication related to the surgery itself, the pain would at least somehow *change*.

Since I had been told that I wouldn't feel better until up to three months after the surgery, by the time the surgery was four months behind me, I knew I should be at least largely recovered. But this wasn't the case. The awful, literal, gut-wrenching pain remained. Every bite of food was painful. My energy level was nonexistent. I even went to work in my pajamas a couple of times to do necessary video editing. When I asked my doctor about the possibility of more diverticulosis, he confirmed my fears by telling me that it was indeed possible that I had more in a different area of my colon. They had taken out the *worst* section of my colon. He assured me that I shouldn't worry about whether there was any more; "at this point it isn't relevant." He again said that there was no preventative measure I could take, the condition was hereditary, and if more of the diverticulosis manifested, we would "cross that bridge when we get there"—even doing additional surgeries if necessary.

All the while, no one in the pharmaceutical, typical Western-medical world suggested I should change my diet. Because of all her research, my wife became increasingly insistent that I might benefit from a more natural diet. At the very least, the two of us were beginning to read some alarming truths about the ingredients in our processed foods. It stood to reason that eliminating those would be a smart move for our children, regardless of whether it helped me. In my attempt to eat cleaner foods, I made such changes as replacing cereals with yogurts and dairies paired with eggs for breakfast. While this was a good step in the right direction, I would later learn that even changes such as these were not enough.

After I should have been fully recovered from my surgery, I was still hurting so badly that I ended up in the ER again. The medics checked my appendix and gallbladder, and even looked at my intestine to make sure there were no collapsed sections, but they simply couldn't find the source of pain. Each time I complained, the aches were explained away as "scar tissue" or "nerve pain." In addition, three months after my surgery, I began to have chest pains so intense that when I went to ER again, the emergency room doctors decided they needed to rule out a possible heart attack. After hours of waiting for basic labs to come back, the doctor came in—by now, it was in the wee hours of the morning—and said, "Joe, I can't tell you that it's your heart, but I can't tell you that it's not, either. We need to run an EKG and echocardiogram, but we can't do that until the cardiologist gets here in the morning."

So, I waited in that emergency room bed all night for the cardiologist. Such a situation gives a man a lot of time to think. I thought about all the times I had worked too many hours instead of spending time with my family and all the times I had underappreciated those dearest to me. I also thought about more than that, particularly how much my illness had stolen from me and my family. I remembered all the kids' basketball games my wife had attended without me, the fun days with the kids at the park that I had missed, and the dates my wife had not been out on because my illness had kept me home. I was sick of this illness and its life-sapping ability to creep in and take from my family, seemingly at its own random and cruel will. I was tired of being weak and missing out on life. That night in that hospital room, I had hours ahead to spend alone (Katherine had to take our newborn home for the night) and wonder what tomorrow would bring. Under the looming suspense of the next morning's tests, I prayed intently that God would help me find a way to break the cycle.

The next morning after the tests results came back, I was both thankful and mystified to learn that my heart was "beautiful." Speculative diagnosis included another bout with pleurisy or stress, and the doctors told me to follow up with my primary care doctor. (This particular ER doctor also recommended that I seek medication for my anxiety.)

Over the last couple of years, I have gotten to know Mark Taylor (the "Fireman Prophet"), and I consider him a close friend. I called him because he has, like me, experienced a lot of ambiguous, hard-to-diagnose medical symptoms. I hoped he could shed some light on the matter. He listened patiently while I described my symptoms, and when I finished, he responded.

"I've been through it, too," he sympathized. "Doctor after doctor, test after test—I know what you're going through, man. And the problem is that if it's not killing you *that day on the gurney*, they really can't diagnose it, for the most part. And, nothing seems very remarkable about most of the symptoms you're describing, because they're so common that they're all pretty much considered normal. I was having pain and anxiety issues because of adrenal burnout from the fire department that I worked at, and I was experiencing all of those symptoms."

Mark then went on to tell me that he had been working with holistic doctors in an attempt to recover from adrenal fatigue, the underlying issue causing many of the symptoms he was having. As I listened to him outline the problems he had experienced throughout the years, a lightbulb went off. And this time, when someone started talking to me about natural remedies, I *listened*.

I began to research holistic remedies, and as I did, I realized that my symptoms connected in a sequence that made sense. A whole new world of understanding opened up to me. I finally started seeing the connection between so many things I had been experiencing over the years, which until now had seemed simultaneous but random: the constant, chronic inflammation throughout my body, the low testosterone, the constant gut pain, the anxiety, the fatty liver, the chest pains, the nausea, and even the tendinitis. Now all these looked very much like they might be connected to the same underlying, deeper condition. Doctors could medicate isolated symptoms all day long, but a further issue within my body had been trying to get my attention, manifesting itself in these other ways.

The colon surgery was successful and effective from a medical standpoint, because it removed the diseased area. Had I continued eating my traditional American diet, the procedure likely would have helped me avoid recurring future intestinal infections. But through my recovery, I realized that all along, despite myriad medical interventions our Western culture has to offer, I had a deeper, underlying problem that could only be addressed through diet and lifestyle. A holistic doctor finally gave me a diagnosis (discussed in more detail in a later chapter) that does not even exist in modern, traditional American medicine: Leaky Gut Syndrome, a disease affecting nearly 80 percent of Americans,[1] although many aren't even aware they are suffering from it! Because the symptoms do not always show up as *actual gut pain*, the surprising truth is that this culprit flies under the radar undetected while it causes or contributes to other, more serious, medical problems. Because of its low-profile characteristic, it goes undiagnosed within the traditional medical world; therefore, its hundreds of side effects, often masquerading as "incurable" chronic illness and other health problems, are all too often treated by addressing *symptoms* and not the *Leaky Gut Syndrome*. You, like me, could be suffering from this culprit and not even realize it! Leaky Gut Syndrome is nothing more than a byproduct of years of engaging in an unhealthy lifestyle and diet, but it shows up in a wide range of chronic illnesses that plague our modern American society, such as chronic fatigue syndrome, rheumatoid arthritis, migraines, fibromyalgia, ulcerative colitis, weight problems, depression, anxiety, lupus, Crohn's disease, irritable bowel syndrome, psoriasis or other rashes, asthma, acquired food allergies, and many other autoimmune or inflammatory diseases. Leaky Gut Syndrome can contribute to diabetes, cancer, heart disease, Alzheimer's disease, Lou Gehrig's disease, Parkinson's disease, and many more illnesses. The gut's importance is often overlooked until it hurts, but this mistake can cost an individual his or her health. Holistic doctors everywhere are emerging with news that connects overall health largely to the gut. Because 70 percent of the immune system's abilities stem from the gut,[2] it is the central force behind our overall well-being and ability to fight illnesses, both serious and not.

I had never had my core, central issue diagnosed and addressed until I went to see my first holistic doctor. And if I had known years ago what I know now, my surgery would have been completely avoidable. I have often said I wish that "Present-Day Joe" could go back twenty years and talk to "Previous-Day Joe" to tell him how to avoid all those years of pain. But of course, hindsight is not reality. However, my own future can be changed, and I hope to help others change theirs by sharing the revelations I've had that affected my health in positive, life-changing ways. As it stands, my follow-up colonoscopy in 2017 after my colon surgery showed no lingering diverticulosis. This means that if I follow "Present-Day Joe's" advice from here on out, I can live free of this illness. I have finally started down a true path to wellness. I'm thrilled and humbled by the progress that I've made since I implemented the lifestyle changes highlighted in this book. Every month has been better. For the first time in over a decade, I have the energy to play chase with my children through the house. My guts are healthier than they've been since childhood, and I'm no longer suffering from irregularity! My brain clarity and ability to focus are no longer hindered by fatigue and sleepiness. I'm not a *hostage* to this chronic illness anymore; *this is the lasting recovery.*

As this new world has opened for me, I've learned a lot about what had been happening throughout my body all those years. I've also met other people who have experienced the same things, all in varying stages of the medical conundrum I'd been in. Some of these folks are only now noticing symptoms, while others have had multiple surgeries and suffer more advanced illness than my own ever became. Not only have I learned how to take charge of my own health through natural healing, I also see how I can help others avoid the same painful and debilitating lifestyle I lived through for so many years. Some people I've talked with are young, and to look at them, you would never suspect that they are suffering with the medical issues that plague them. Before more serious health issues arise for these individuals, it's my goal to intervene and keep them from going down the road that I lived on for so long.

I have been asked why I would write a book that discloses so many personal and intimate details of my challenges with health after so many years of keeping them from public view. In addition to being encouraged to do so by my family, I think about if one of my children was suffering with a chronic illness. If someone out there had been through the same or similar journey and possibly held the key to helping one of my kids find healing, I would want that person to intervene and share that knowledge with us. Frankly, I am so excited about the healing I've received that keeping it to myself seems self-indulgent, when I know people right now could be living a higher-quality life but have been *conditioned to believe otherwise*. But this type of thinking is part of the problem. We have to adjust our perspective. I spent years thinking that I was looking for a path *back* to wellness. But *back* is the wrong direction. *Back* returns me and my family to old habits such as pizza nights and banana-split Sundays. The key is to walk *away* from all those routines and into a new life. We must make it a lifestyle to leave those behaviors behind—once and for all—and move forward into a new lifestyle of balance and health in order to care for our bodies as a whole. The answer is not to move *back* to health, but to move *forward into our healing* by changing our lifestyle.

The issues I will address in this book affect everybody; disease is on the rise. The number of people diagnosed with cancer, high blood pressure, diabetes, and other increasingly common diseases seem to be at all-time highs. Obesity, a gateway to other, more serious problems for many individuals, is a rising epidemic across our country. The cost of healthcare is escalating and creating an enormous impact on our economy. Pinpointing the cause of such issues can cause an ambiguous debate that results in much finger-pointing. When it comes right down to it, everybody knows that everyone *else* should be taking better care of their health. Many of us think we can look around and identify those with health issues at a glance, but, as my story indicates, that's not always possible. I was very sick for many years, and only my closest friends and family knew there was even a problem.

Through this experience, I gained more understanding of what's really happening behind the scenes regarding our current society's health epidemic. With guidance from healthcare professionals who educated me and put me on the natural path to health, I've set out on a new mission to learn all I can about our modern American diet, our common health issues, and the relationship between the two. With each layer I have peeled back, I've discovered new information just beneath it that has been even more startling. The rabbit hole, at times, seems bottomless.

In the movie *The Matrix*, a character named Cypher says, "Why, oh why, didn't I take the blue pill?"[3] after choosing to enlighten himself to the truth as to what the Matrix truly was. At times in my journey, that's been me. Once I began to learn about our modern American food supply and how it is impacting our health, the more overwhelming it has been at times. It is staggering to realize how much we need to change about our products industries, and simultaneously how outnumbered and small we are as single consumers.

However, there is good news. *We, as consumers, also have the power to make a change.* When *we* are holding our money, *we* are ultimately in control. When *we* prepare our meals, *we* are filtering what we put into our bodies. When *we* supplement our food with additional vitamins and nutrients, *we* are ensuring our nutritional intake, despite compromised nutritional content of food. It's easy to feel outnumbered and powerless. It's even easier to become frustrated when we feel like we are gaining ground, only to have a label change or some other marketing scheme pull the rug from under us, leaving us feeling again as though some grand "reset" button has sent us back to square one.

But there is encouragement: Conglomerates are losing sales rapidly on many junk foods, causing an increasing presence of labels like "organic" and "natural" on the grocery store shelves. Farm-to-fork movements are on the rise, organic farmers are uniting to expose labeling fraud, and we, the American population in general, are increasingly attempting to educate ourselves about what we are eating. The fruits of these laborers are beginning to show up everywhere: Even large fast-food chains like McDonalds are now advertising that they *intend* to go organic within a certain number of years.

While this is good news, it raises nearly as many questions as answers. Can we trust food labeling? What does the "organic" label mean? Can we really make a difference in what our families are eating with limited time and on a budget? These questions and so many more often leave people mentally frozen and unsure what direction to move, until their own insecurity slowly drives them back into the comfort zone of die-hard, nutritionally bankrupt dietary habits.

The battle is not yet won, but we're at a place where a transition can begin. I discovered with my own health that my problem was twofold. Part of the problem was ignorance and possibly even complacency about what I *was* putting into my body, and the other was the lack of supplementation and other natural, preventative intervention toward the benefit of health.

This is how I believe my story can help you. While it is still being written, after fifteen years of living with debilitating illness, I've entered a chapter of true and sustainable healing. The changes I have made—both what I've *eliminated from* my life and what I've *added to* my life—can encourage and steer you, I hope, by demystifying the process of finding safe and healthy foods for you and your family. In a later chapter, I will share more about the *specific steps* that were vital to regaining my own health, the specifics of my diagnosis and its symptoms, and how to begin the reversal process.

This is not a cookbook, a fad-diet endorsement, or quick-fix nutrition plan. It is the accumulation of research into the cutting-edge discoveries linking our toxic, modern-American food supply to the current public health crisis. As brought forth by holistic doctors and scientists worldwide, this timely material has been compiled into a format that will empower you to prevent unnecessary disease, untangle the confusing advertising structure of the food conglomerates, avoid the most common disease-creating toxins being smuggled into your food every day, and help you identify the tricks employed in modern food-labeling schemes. If you're one of the millions of Americans experiencing any of the symptoms listed earlier in this chapter, you could already be carrying the timebomb. Even if you currently believe you're in great health and eating a proper diet, this book reveals how you might still unknowingly be eating foods that are detrimental to your long-term well-being and uncovers what you can do about it. Time is ticking. Keep reading... It's time to see beyond the corporate smokescreen and reclaim the health of yourself and your children.

2

Change Your Frame of Mind

The average American citizen races through daily life at what seems like the speed of light. We wake up, down a cup of coffee, and grab a snack that we call breakfast (if we're lucky enough to remember breakfast at all) before hurrying off to work at high stress levels until noon. Once our lunch break has begun, we dart erratically across town, running errands while scarfing a burger and fries that we scarf down with a super-sized soda. When the lunch hour is over, we breathlessly return to our stress-infused jobs in workplaces that are often illuminated by only artificial light. There we spend the rest of the afternoon until it is time once again to pile into the car and traverse through gridlocked traffic amid road-raged antagonists until we finally arrive home. Before our next round of duties—kids' homework, laundry, taxes, bills—we cook a "home-made" meal of Hamburger Helper, mac & cheese, or some other prefabricated food and wash it down with a healthier drink than our lunchtime option, such as Gatorade or fruit juice. (After all, we're at home with the kids now, and we wouldn't want them eating the way we did at lunch, so we go the extra mile for them by cooking and avoiding soft drinks.) Before bed, we enjoy some sort of indulgence such as ice cream, a sugary dessert, or possibly even candy.

This is a normal scenario in our society. I know this because I was guilty of this routine for years! At this point, the reader may retort that people are doing this because they're not being prudent about their health, or because they don't care. These people are often written off as careless with their own health and the health of their children. But let's set that reaction aside for a moment and take a closer look at our society's habits. What is the real motivation behind our continued poor eating habits? Many of us are aware that we're eating unhealthy food. Yet we have somehow been lulled into complacency about the subject. Why?

The answer can be as varied as we are: the expense of eating organic foods, the lack of time it takes to prepare healthy meals, not knowing the basics of good nutrition, or even an attitude summed up in the adage: "Life is short; eat dessert first—you only live once!"

Most Americans don't judge each other for living this way; it seems like the machinations of our modern lifestyle have simply turned, landing us all at a point where this is all we feel we have time for. Many parents, trying to do their very best for their children, look at this picture and feel dividedly remorseful. On one hand, they admit that this portrayal matches up with an average day in their life, yet they are simultaneously rueful that they can't be more proactive about their children's health. I know several parents who admit that the food their children are eating is not ideal, but between working full time and juggling the many responsibilities of life, they feel powerless to take control of the situation. One working mother teasingly said to me recently (while shrugging off the apparent hopelessness that had pressed her into submission): "I don't have time to become some rocket-scientist-health-guru-organic chef!" It's an understandable dilemma.

I would wager that part of the issue at the core of our complacency is that we don't realize how dangerous our food is. To people who haven't taken the time to learn about what they're putting into their bodies, the idea of our food being substandard is an ambiguous, looming cloud of vagueness over our heads that we know may someday catch up with us. But as long as the byproducts of such unhealthy habits do not manifest themselves in the form of symptoms or illnesses, we continue to deal with our "more immediate needs"—the demands of daily life—hoping that sometime soon we will finally have the "time and resources" to tackle the issue of our food.

If only the average consumers truly understood how dangerous their food is, they might consider it a more immediate need to address the threat of our diets. When we are aware of a fire hazard in our house such as faulty wiring, we don't ignore it for years until the house finally catches fire. If our vehicle shows signs of an issue with brakes or steering, we take it to a shop for repair. Any time we see impending danger, we address it. So, when it comes to food, our lack of awareness of the important issues involving it is where the biggest danger comes in. We wouldn't be so complacent if we understood how far down the rabbit hole goes.

Notable about this subject is that, as consumers, our greatest weakness—lack of knowledge—can also become a strength. Once we change the way we *think* about food, then we can meet the seduction of advertising, the trap of complacency, and the hopelessness of confusion with recognition and resistance. The antidote to the absence of knowledge is *education*. Knowledge is power. Consumers are not without power. We just have to learn how to take it back. Once we've done so, we can find healthy food for our families no matter how much junk floods into the marketplace.

A Cornucopia of Gray Matter

Since you are reading this book, it is possible that you weren't alive in the early 1900s, when the average woman spent forty-four hours per week in the kitchen[4] preparing all meals from scratch. In the 1950s, time spent preparing the family's meals had decreased to twenty hours per week.[5] In the present-day household, women (or men) average less than ten hours per week on food preparation and cleanup, with some clocking no time at all on food prep. On top of this, 44 percent of the money spent on food today is done so at restaurants![6] The statistics for the younger generations are even more shocking: The average Millennial spends less than twenty minutes a day on food prep and doesn't even know how to cook.[7] The irony is that as our confidence in, interest in, or ability to prepare our own meals has declined, our kitchens have become larger, more glamorous, and better equipped than ever.

Many households don't have even one member who knows how to cook without the aid of a pre-boxed meal kit. *Huffington Post* recently reported that 28 percent of Americans don't know how to cook,[8] while other studies, such as a recent one conducted by the Department of Health, shows that only one in six mothers makes a meal from scratch each day[9].

We as a society have let our guard down concerning food. Advertising now appeals to our emotional mind, instead of our practical mind. Doctors (or actors portraying doctors) wearing lab coats endorse the healthy attributes of particular foods, and words and phrases like "natural" and "no sugar added" are tossed out like a safety net to persuade trusting shoppers to purchase the least of all evils for their families. Consumers cling to the hope that "they" ("they" being a higher power governing food safety on behalf of the consumer, which we will discuss in another chapter) are vetting the products on the market and scrutinizing everything that is sold with tight safety standards.

Is the modern consumer tricked? Those of us who aren't fooled into believing our food is healthy, as stated before, might say we don't have time to address the issue. Others, because of our lack of knowledge, feel helpless and simply shrug off the problem, hoping they will be among the lucky few who dodge the bullet that is the food they're eating. Yet others laugh and pretend they don't care—and maybe they really don't. Such an apathetic stance is also a direct response to the core problem. But, we are intelligent, educated people, right? We have all the tools available, we have the big kitchens, we are surrounded by "food," and are generally a bright, progressive generation. We rally about, advocating for human rights, the environment, endangered species, religious world views, and any other causes we feel are worth protecting. So why not speak out about the health of our bodies? Why not advocate for our right to healthy food choices? *Just what is the underlying problem?*

Again, I don't believe most of us understand exactly what we're putting into our bodies and how dangerous most of those foods and drinks are. We watch with vigilance for *obvious* enemies. But much of what we eat is an enemy invader waging war on our immune systems and affecting our bodies. And, when is an enemy ever intentionally obvious? Stealth is all too often used by an enemy as a tactical advantage. When you look around your environment for the enemy, you're probably not thinking about checking your cabinets. Like many, you're probably looking for *obvious* combatants—illegal drugs, alcohol, even tobacco products—while the seemingly safe food in your kitchen is likely more toxic than you know.

The Timely and the Convenient

Allow me to turn to a mythological tale that presents a useful analogy in many Americans' views about the food we eat. Legend has it that the Greek god Caerus, son of Zeus, was noted for the single lock of hair atop his head. The only way to catch this god, as mythology has it, was by gripping this lock of hair as he headed toward you. Once he had passed you, there was no catching him, as his backside had nothing to grab. Those hoping to catch him had to see him coming, clutch that lock of hair, and hang on before their chance was gone.

Caerus was the god of opportunity, bringing about what was "just in time and convenient," as the legends say. His was the way of last-minute convenience. He was beautiful to look at, always on tiptoe, and had wings on his feet for the swift movement in flight. He was also known to show volatile, hostile behavior toward humans, and was often even said to have drunk their blood.

Consider the parallels between this ancient Greek entity and our society's affinity toward anything that requires minimal effort. Favorable, easy opportunity, in a swift and timely fashion, holds a very attractive seduction for us in our hurried lifestyles. Many of us move throughout our day, racing at the mercy of everything that comes at the last minute and through expedience. We move as if we believe we had wings on our own feet, but perhaps we are really dancing with an entity that would drink our blood.

Am I saying that by driving through a fast-food restaurant for a cheeseburger, we're worshiping Caerus, son of Zeus? I wouldn't go *that far*. But I *am* saying that just like Caerus, we must identify and seize the problem rapidly approaching us, because it is an entity that offers convenience, but it is hostile (even blood-drinking) to humans. We only have a certain amount of time to reach up, grab that lock of hair, and hang on tight, putting up a fight for our safety. Once the opportunity to fight for our well-being has passed (and on his backside, we have nothing to grip), no method of subduing the enemy is available. This could leave us having missed our opportunity for change, and we could be left with diabetes, cancer, or some other kind of illness that is potentially irreversible.

The Worst Ingredient in Our Food

The point that I am trying to drive home comes down to this: The worst ingredient in our food is our complacency toward it. The first toxic thing we put on our plate is our lackadaisical attitude about the next thing we put on our plate: our food.

So, now that I have made this point abundantly clear, how do we go about changing this first dangerous ingredient? Where did this ingredient even come from? And how do we proceed?

Recall the scenario highlighted earlier in the book of the average American racing through the day at light speed. This person (and it's probably nearly everyone: you, me, your Aunt Nancy, and my neighbor Sam) has justifiable reasons for wanting to breeze through mealtime and move on to the next chapter of his or her day. The cycle that perpetuates throughout our day, linking one "whirlwind" activity to the next, creates a place in which it's hard to even identify where the problem begins and where it ends. How we arrived at this point, and where to initiate the first steps of change, become conversations that begin to sound like the proverbial "chicken and the egg" conversation. For example:

Having a journal can help you organize your time, but I doubt you are keeping a journal, even though it would help you account for how you are spending your time. On the other hand, if you had the time to keep a journal, you likely would have already organized your time.

If you felt you could afford to eat healthier food, you might already be doing so. So, by avoiding the extra expense now, you are likely making a trade that will result in doctor bills later if they are not already stacking up. Many people know this, but recognizing this as a dilemma and knowing how to break out of it are two very different things.

These cyclical patterns feed themselves and are difficult to disrupt. When I was in grade school and the kids used to jump rope, we would use a very long rope. One child on each end would "twirl" the rope. The children about to jump in would hold their hands, palms out, in front of their chest, mimicking the placement of the rope. This hand motion would help them to get a feel for the rhythm of the rope as it rotated in front of them, until they had a good enough handle on its timing to jump in. They would then jump into the middle of the rope, and continue jumping until they missed, when they were given one end of the rope to become the new "twirler." Then, the next child in line would take a turn jumping.

The trick for these children was standing in front of the rope before they jumped in, calculating the rhythm. They assessed for a moment, deciding how to insert themselves into the cycle of the rope so they could jump within the rhythm as it rotated around them. It didn't always work on the first try. But anyone who kept trying got it eventually.

However, it took finding that starting point, when they could jump in while the rope was still moving. That is much like what we must do regarding our current food cycle: stand back, assess the situation, find a place we think is a good starting point, and jump in.

Psychology of the Shopper

As I've already stated, the first dangerous ingredient in our food is our attitude toward it. By this, I'm obviously also saying we need to gain a new perspective regarding our food. It seems the best place to start is at the beginning: the place where we obtain our food. For most of us, this would be local chain grocery store; for the sake of relating to the average consumer, this is where I will begin this leg of our journey.

Consider average shoppers, who are balancing all the responsibilities of daily life. Take a moment to relate to what is happening in their minds. How do they select purchases for their families? What criteria factor into getting an item off the shelf and into their shopping carts?

Many of us don't even realize that the scene has been set long before we even lay eyes on the food for sale in these places. Think about it: When you walk into a grocery store, you usually enter through the produce department. These displays feature the freshest of all the ingredients in the store. You're immediately surrounded by products that appear to be garden fresh, and your line of vision is immediately flooded with overhanging, billboard-sized pictures of food that looks fresh, healthy, and appetizing.

The produce department sits beneath these larger-than-life images displaying fresh-cut tomatoes of only the highest quality, placed directly beside succulent cuts of the greenest broccoli. Nearby might hang another photo of lettuce, freshly pulled from the garden and so recently rinsed that its leaves are still wet. Moving farther into the grocery store, you'll see that over the meat department hovers a picture depicting fresh, lean cuts of only the pinkest prime meat. Over the dairy section…well… you get the picture.

These signs present subliminal messages that say, "You have entered an arena of food that is healthy, fresh, and safe. You are in a trustworthy zone for making excellent purchases for your family." Your mind adopts these images as an unspoken standard, which you then subliminally presume applies to other items in the store. When you round the corner aisle and the smell of the deli's precooked rotisserie chicken hits your nostrils, you unknowingly carry the sense of security generated in the produce department over to that product. You start rethinking your previous plan of stopping for pizza on the way home. Your mind might say, "This is healthy. In fact, how can you *get any healthier* than a whole chicken? And this is already cooked for me. It's been a long day. Instead of having a pizza, I'll make the healthy decision. I'll take one of those home to my family." After turning another corner, perhaps you find yourself looking at shelves of soup. The pictures on the can labels show steamy, whole vegetables piled up in an earthy, ceramic bowl from amid chunks of meat in a broth flecked with lentils or barley. The very image suggests comfort and peace on a rainy day. You might then think, "I should pick up some of this soup. It's a healthy option for lunches, and it's good to have around if someone gets a cold or flu."

Perhaps you now head down a different aisle, one more colorful than the previous few. Bold colors and advertising language seem to fly off the packaging of cookies, crackers, chips, and other snacks, promising "fun, full flavor" and excitement. Some have the word "WIN" in all capitals in a corner, where details of a sweepstakes of some sort appear below in a smaller font. Trusted childhood friends, those popular cartoon characters children spend so many hours with, appear on much of the packaging, inviting kids to indulge and parents to endorse. "After all," one might think, "if Casey the Clown taught my child on Saturday morning that stealing is wrong, surely she's a wholesome role model for which snacks to eat as well, right?"

When you see the bright red and orange packaging (colors scientifically found to rouse hunger[10]) splashed with images of young, teenaged boys having an adventurous time on a mountain bike or a skateboard, you might be intrigued by the excitement suggested on the packaging and think, "That looks like fun. I'll bet the kids would really enjoy these. I'll just get one or two bags to treat them with. After all, they are such good kids and they deserve a treat." At this point, you're more aware that what you're purchasing isn't healthy, but you justify it by thinking, "The *rest* of what I'm buying is healthy." Unfortunately, what you've done, without even realizing it, is embrace an unspoken message sent by the images that surrounded you within your first moments inside the supermarket. These images, which you unknowingly adopted, caused you to espouse a "safe" feeling that you have now applied, ever-changing as it may be from item to item, throughout the entire store. That standard of quality, however, was derived from a quick glance at something as simple as a picture of a sliced tomato and wet lettuce, and was presumed within *your own mind;* it is not guaranteed *anywhere* within the store.

As you progress through the store, you apply the self-implied safety standard to more and more of the products until, inch by inch, you've covered the entire store and made selections from each aisle. The appealing images of groceries are placed strategically to coerce you into feeling at peace with the items in front of them on the shelf. It makes sense: You buy when you feel safe, and the hidden messaging that greets you at the door can carry its rationale through all the decisions you have made until you are loading the groceries into the trunk of your car and then driving home to feed it all to your family.

Fixing That First Ingredient

As stated before, the most dangerous ingredient in our food is our attitude toward it. When that changes, we can begin to make progress. We have to undo what brought us to the point we're at in order for this to happen. Part of the solution is to face that we have been seduced over time by complacency, exhaustion, and the urge for convenience in a world that keeps us busy. But, there's another angle we need to explore.

Food is not emotional, nor is it entertaining. Advertising is.

Advertising schemes promoting all sorts of products—not just food and beverages—often appeal to the emotions to generate sales. Revisit your walk through the grocery store outlined in the last few paragraphs. The soup appealed to your need for comfort and peace, while the snack selection charmed you with promises of fun and excitement with trusted "friends," such as the aforementioned Casey the Clown. We humans are wired to want these things. In that way, it is natural to assume that the products promising such benefits are the products toward which we migrate. But how many consumers give this matter any thought? How many realize the basis for their decisions? Who is analyzing the criteria that decides their purchases? As stated before, this is a *subliminal* lure, which means that many don't even see the path our thoughts are taking when we make our purchases. Have you ever considered *why* you're drawn to the foods that tempt you when you're shopping? It might go something like this:

That soup looks warm and delicious. Life was hard today. I want that soup to make me feel better.

-or-

I'm bored. Those chips look fun. So do these cookies.

-or-

I feel lonely and neglected. This "indulgent, luxurious" chocolate looks seductive.

But herein lies so much of our problem. We want *food* to make us *feel better*. We want food to supplement the satisfaction we're not getting from a dead-end job or the fun missing from a lackluster social life. Worst of all, the food is making us feel *worse* (more on this later). On top of that, when we gain weight because of the food choices we're making, many of us withdraw, keeping further to ourselves…and that feeds into our disappointment with our social lives which lowers our performance at work. See the cycle? It's only one of many wrapped up in the complicated subject of our food.

Adjusting Our Thinking

Food is fuel. This is a simple fact. We absolutely *have to* let go of the tendency to link our food with our emotional experience. Think about it this way: If your body was a machine and required batteries, hydraulic fluids, and certain amounts of lubricating oils at specific maintenance intervals, would you put more of these products in it than necessary? I doubt you would add foreign substances that weren't on the maintenance instructions, just for "fun" or for any other reason connected to emotions. You would likely presume that doing so would interfere with the machine's operations. Our bodies are no different. We need a certain amount of nutrition at intervals that create our optimal performance. Another complication is the foreign substances we regularly put into our bodies. That causes us to suffer, to become "out of whack," just as a machine would do under similar circumstances.

We also need to change our ideas about food being instant. That's not to say there isn't "instant food," but typically, those products have no nutritional value. Worse, many are loaded with toxic ingredients (this will be outlined in a later chapter). Since the introduction of processed food, our disease rates have skyrocketed. Whether we realize it or not, this is another byproduct of our complacency toward food. You might think I'm being harsh, but I don't mean to be. I'm not saying this from a place of judgment (remember, I have spent the last fifteen years dealing with chronic illness); I just know that many people don't realize how harmful these processed foods are. When we emotionally separate ourselves from our food, we realize what our food is *not*. Next, we must rethink what our food *is*. We must remember its *purpose*. When we emphasize that food is fuel for our bodies and not entertainment or emotional satisfaction, we'll adjust our priorities accordingly. And when this happens, we'll realize that it *is possible* to create more time in our schedule for proper nutrition. We'll begin to safeguard with more diligence what we are buying, and we'll discover ways to afford better food. We will change our expectations of the finished product and be satisfied with food in its nutritious simplicity.

Feeling Overwhelmed Yet?

If you feel tempted to put down the book and return to old habits at this point, I understand. But before you do, I urge you to remember that this would likely be an emotional reaction founded in fear and lack of confidence, as this broad subject, as stated previously, can easily become overwhelming. Your health and the health of your children could depend on whether you keep reading. It is understandable if feeling overwhelmed tempts you to decide not to think about this enormous issue. Believe me, I've been there, and there is hope! I, for example, was the last person anyone ever expected to learn how to cook, plan meals, or stick to a specific meal structure. However, my health eventually declined to the point that my diet demanded my attention, regardless of what I may have perceived my priorities to be. Now I prepare nearly all my family's meals and have really learned to love reading labels and knowing what we put into our bodies. I now find joy in cooking! That transformation highlights the purpose of this book: to shed light on a path that was shadowed in confusion when I was on my journey, and to simplify the transition for the reader.

I challenge you to take charge of your situation: Learn how to become your own vigilant guard. If you try, you can take the emotion out of the equation and begin to make purchases based on the principle that the food you eat is fuel. You are your primary advocate. As a wise consumer, you can be part of the solution. You're not powerless, and you don't have to be a rocket-scientist-health-guru-organic chef to change the way you and your family eat. In this book, we will discuss the dangers in your food, how to watch the ingredients on your food labels, and how to use your money to cast your ballot·each time you shop. The transitions you make can be gradual. This doesn't need to happen overnight. On the contrary, if you are the type of person who has trouble following through when a change has been made too suddenly, then I encourage you to approach this process more slowly. The important thing is to take steps toward your goal. If you're determined, you can, even on a shoestring budget and with a cramped schedule, begin to overhaul your family's eating habits.

There are forces that want you to close this book. Like Cipher from *The Matrix,* choosing to swallow the pill that would allow him to go back into a false sense of reality where his life is not his own, but where he is more comfortable, you may find yourself wishing you had taken the other pill. My illness did not allow me that luxury. I hope you'll never find yourself at the point I reached. I pray that you will take this information and use it as a critical preventative measure for yourself and your family. If you're already ill, then believe me when I tell you that I've learned firsthand that chronic illness often can be reversed, once you eliminate from your lifestyle the things that are making you sick and introduce good things that your body needs to heal.

I implore you as a responsible individual, and as one who presumably values your health, as a concerned member of a society being kept sick by conspiracies that line the pockets of the wealthy elite (more on this later), or even as a parent: Please don't put this book down and go back to your old habits. Knowledge is power, and by the time you reach the end of this book, you'll understand how to reclaim yours.

3

Uncovering the Conspiracy

Before moving forward in our subject of food, chronic illness, and dietary issues, I would like to discuss some parallels found within the tobacco industry. Allow me to recall a time when cigarettes seemed harmless. Smoking was "cool," and everybody who was anybody did it. In movies, even doctors sitting at their desks *in hospitals* were seen smoking! In the early 1960s, *The Flintstones* cartoon series was sponsored by Winston cigarettes, which ran the famous ad campaign, "Winston tastes good like a cigarette should."[11]

Fast-forward fifty years, and we see that the attitude toward tobacco changed significantly. What was once regarded as a fairly harmless activity has now been revealed to be the deadly habit that it is. In March of 2012, Dr. Margaret Chan, director-general of the World Health Organization, in a keynote address at the 15th World Conference on Tobacco or Health in Singapore, stated the following:

> This conference is being held at a time when we are at a crossroads in our efforts to rid the world of a killing addiction. In principle, the balance is entirely in our favor. In a perfectly sane, reasonable, rational world, with a level playing field, the anti-

tobacco community would surely speak with the loudest voice and carry the biggest stick.

Evidence for the physical harm, and economic costs, of tobacco use keeps growing.… We know that tobacco directly harms the user's health in multiple ways. We know that tobacco products kill their consumers. We know that tobacco smoking, like a drive–by shooting, kills innocent bystanders who are forced to breathe air contaminated with hundreds of toxic chemicals. We know what tobacco exposure during pregnancy does to the fetus, another innocent, blameless, and entirely helpless victim.

We know that tobacco use is not a choice. It is a powerful addiction. The true choice is between tobacco or health.[12]

What changed over fifty years? Awareness, public outcry, and eventually changes in legislation caused bans to be placed on when and how tobacco could be marketed, determined who the target audiences could be, and implemented the requirement for warning labels on products to increase the buyers' awareness of the dangers of tobacco use. It is now common knowledge that tobacco products are killing more than five million people per year.[13] The risks and effects of smoking, both to the user and to those around them, have been disclosed to the public. Workplaces have either designated specific areas for smoking or declared that they are completely tobacco-free facilities. Pregnant women have been made aware of the risks that smoking cigarettes present to their unborn children. The dangers of secondhand smoke have been brought to the attention of parents. Programs designed to help smokers "kick the habit" are available at little or no cost in communities everywhere. The list of changes in attitudes toward and policies about tobacco use goes on and on, and it all started with people who identified a public health risk and took a stand against it.

Now that the tobacco industry has been properly demonized and such products are no longer associated with such influential characters as those found on our kids' favorite cartoons, we may not be surprised that the advertising industry has moved into using beloved animated characters to promote and endorse another dangerous addiction—children's snacks: cereals, crackers, cookies, and more.

The tobacco industry spent a lot of time dodging the real debate and paying scientists to claim their products were not dangerous. Eventually, however, the truth prevailed, and healthy changes began to take place. We are in a similar revolution now, with food at the center of the upheaval—but it cannot take place unless we are willing to fight. The longer we stand by and allow toxic foods to be marketed to our children, the more lives will be destroyed and lost. But, like those who fought for transparency regarding the risks of tobacco use, we can take a stand and push for changes in our food industry for the improvement of overall public health.

Where Is the FDA in All This?

By this time, we have made our point that most people feel their resources of time and money are spread too thin in one way or another to address the issue of diet. We've made a case for the psychological side of a shopper's series of choices. But there is still a deeper problem that goes hand in hand with that first toxic ingredient in our food—our attitude toward it. This is the fact that when we have exhausted our own efforts, we often rest in the false sense of security that there is an agency looking out for our best interests.

This is what causes many people to fall into the trap of hoping that a greater power is watching, regulating the food we purchase, and vetting out anything that isn't safe to be consumed. For many, the mind reverts to those impressive visual banners hanging in the grocery store displaying the fresh food. Surely a benevolent power out there is regulating what is put into these arenas of food marketing. After all, where else would all this healthy food have come from? These officers act as our "protectors," watching how produce is grown, how bread is baked, how nutrition labels are worded. "They" are believed by many people to act as a dietary guardian angel. People confidently believe that what is approved by the FDA falls under an umbrella of safety.

Because it does… Right?

Wrong.

You might be thinking: "Surely the FDA would never allow sales of dangerous substances. Why would it allow unsafe items to be sold to the American public?" The speculations as to why the answer to this question might be "yes" would fill another book, so I won't go into that here. Instead, I'll outline some of the history surrounding the introduction of GMO (genetically modified organisms) foods into the market. The Flavr Savr tomato case discussed in upcoming pages is one of many that shows the FDA is either overwhelmed, ambivalent, or nefarious (the reader may decide) in its operations. Regardless of the reasoning behind the FDA's actions, it remains true that lethal ingredients, substances, and drugs are approved every day by the FDA. If you have trouble believing this, do a little bit of research on any common medication that comes to mind. A simple Google search of side effects of most common drugs quickly reveals that the substances are often as deadly as they are helpful. Food ingredients bring up an equal list of concerns—and, unlike prescription drugs, these elements aren't even sold with a promise of somehow being medically beneficial. These risky food ingredients are merely added for flavor, visual effect, or preservation.

By the FDA's own admission, it is unable to inspect most of the food imported to the United States. A report pulled from the official FDA website begins with the following:

> FDA has the resources to inspect only a handful of foreign facilities, and physically examines less than 1% of shipments offered for import. FDA uses a risk–based prediction algorithms to prioritize inspections.[14]

Later in the report, the FDA admits it "does not randomly sample import shipments for inspection." The report also explains that the risk-based prediction algorithm in place helps flag areas that may be bringing in problem products, thus prompting a subsequent inspection by the FDA. Inspections that result in refused shipments often are done so due to sanitary violations, unsafe pesticide residues, or the presence of salmonella bacteria. Another main culprit for refused shipments is "misbranding, which may include untruthful or misleading labels or labels that lack English." The three countries that receive the most refusals by the FDA are Mexico, India, and China. Of these countries, the report states that "the persistence of the same problems, year after year, in food import shipments indicates that FDA's inspection regime has not completely deterred producers and importers from offering food shipments for import that violate US laws."

By the FDA's own admission, "the nonrandom nature of FDA sampling means that researchers cannot draw inferences about the relative safety of food produced in various countries or the relative risk of certain food products."[15]

The point I am trying to make is that even if no conspiracy is involved (the reader may believe there *is* a conspiracy by the end of this book), by the FDA's own admission, it is overwhelmed and simply *cannot* be everywhere, watching everything at the same time.

Responsibility for our purchases and their nutritional properties ultimately falls on each of us. There is no "they" to protect us. Even purchasing from "nutritional" brands can be a slippery slope, as most are indeed owned by the larger food conglomerates. The illusion that there is an agency watching out for us, vetting the selections and acting as a discriminating gatekeeper for what is sold beneath the pictures of the garden-fresh, dripping lettuce in the produce section, is exactly that: an illusion.

The Flavr Savr Tomato

In the 1990s, Calgene Inc. introduced the first genetically engineered tomato: the Flavr Savr. This tomato took eight years and more than $20 million to bring about. Unlike previous tomatoes on the market, this new and improved tomato was designed to be picked ripe and last longer in this ripened state. Before now, tomatoes had been picked when they were green. Then they were shipped and treated to prompt ripening just before being displayed for sale in the stores. This industry practice prevented the stocking of soft, overripe, and "squishy" tomatoes on supermarket shelves.

The Flavr Savr's "softening gene" essentially had been disabled, resulting in a tomato that could be left on the vine until ripe, but would still stay firm throughout the shipping process.

When the new product was released, Calgene responded to potential consumer concerns by labeling the tomatoes as a GMO product and even included an 800 number for calls with inquiries about GMO products. Calgene voluntarily underwent the FDA approval process for this tomato in an effort to be transparent and gain and maintain consumer confidence.

During the FDA investigation, Calgene conducted three twenty-eight-day studies, which involved feeding the Flavr Savr to lab rats. To conduct this study, two separate but identical lines of the Flavr Savr tomato were created for the purpose of comparison to each other in a controlled experimental setting.

Both lines included the same gene inserted into the same type of tomato. It is necessary to understand that the process of inserting the gene, followed by the cloning of the cell into the plant, can cause unique results each time, due to slight variations within the gene insertion and cloning procedure at the time it is conducted. This means the scientist can follow the same procedure multiple times, using the same materials, the same tools, and the same methods, yet end up with varying results.

When the first study was conducted, each of the two engineered lines of the tomato was fed separately to two sample populations of twenty lab rats each. Researchers observed the rats for reactions to the specific tomato line that had been created and then fed to them.

Initial reports showed that the twenty rats fed one of the engineered lines of tomato didn't suffer any adverse effects. Of the rats fed the other type of tomato, however, seven of the twenty developed bleeding stomach lesions and tumors, and some died.

These labs, which performed these tests at Calgene's expense, noted that the results manifested possible "treatment-related" problems due to the appearance of the bleeding stomach lesions. Scientists within the FDA acknowledged that the tomatoes failed to exhibit "reasonable certainty of no harm," which is the normal standard of safety determined by the FDA.

The media blitz around the tomato was controversial: Some stories showed people proudly tasting the tomatoes and professing their confidence in the product, unfazed by the GMO status. Others were dubious.

Argument in favor of the tomato's approval was often heavily formulated around the emphasis that there was no scientific basis proving the tomato was unsafe. Arguments against the approval of the tomato and other incoming GMO foods dubbed them as "scientifically unfounded." The issue was simply that no science existed on the products at all because they were brand new. The FDA's official statement was that it would ensure that the biotech products were treated with the same safety oversight as other foods, without being hampered by unnecessary regulation. As a precaution, Calgene destroyed the line that had caused stomach lesions in the experiment subjects.

When Calgene repeated the study, feeding the Flavr Savr tomato to thirty-five rats this time, there were only three casualties. During this testing, the tomatoes were administered in a freeze-dried form, allowing scientists to place the concentrated tomato into each subject.

Willing to acknowledge that unresolved questions lingered, the FDA was pressed with the question: To approve or not to approve? It swept concerns regarding the tomato under the rug and deemed the tomato safe. But alas, Calgene openly admitted that while its scientists were trying to create a better food source, they were not skilled as agricultural grocery distributors. On the distribution end, they made so many mistakes that they couldn't turn a profit with the new product. Eventually, Calgene was bought out by Monsanto. But if this tomato wasn't profitable, why did Monsanto purchase the company? Could it be that Monsanto was trying to silence a competitor that was interested in transparency? The tomato has been removed from shelves, and the only place that the Flavr Savr tomato seed can be found today is in a Monsanto vault. Why? Could it be because Calgene had patents on key technology and Monsanto was anxious to eliminate a competitor who was calling for appropriate labeling and was dedicated to the kind of transparency that Monsanto wasn't comfortable with? And, since Calgene was bought out by Monsanto, no GMO food manufacturer has been so forthcoming with research regarding its product and given such detailed reports as these to this day.

A Further Investigation...

Dr. Arpad Pusztai, a scientist, nutritionist, biochemist, and molecular biologist, was one of the first to voice concerns about safety as it pertains to GMO foods. He spent thirty-six years at the Rowett Research Institute in Aberdeen, Scotland, until statements about the negative effects of GMO foods on lab rats resulted in criticism and eventual suspension from his position there. Of the gene-insertion process, he said:

> Gene insertion is a major problem. You cannot direct where the splicing of the genetic construct will happen. It is well-

known that when you insert a genetic construct into the DNA network of a plant, you create changes in that network. As a result, you will get changes in the functionality of the plants own genes. They may become more active or silent. The effects will be unpredictable and uncontrollable. It can sometimes cause irreparable damage to the genome. This is insertional mutagenesis.[16]

This is the same type of process that would have been used in engineering the Flavr Savr tomato. When Dr. Pusztai reviewed the lab documents from the Flavr Savr tomato, he found many discrepancies within the initial report.

What actually happened during the testing? The feedings were conducted in three twenty-eight-day segments. Allow me to recall your attention to the fact that two types of tomatoes were created for this experiment. The rats eating one of the types remained healthy and seemed to show no adverse effects.

Dr. Pusztai had many concerns about the other type when reviewing these documents. The FDA's explanation for the rats that died of bleeding stomach lesions was that these issues were caused by mucolytic agents in the tomatoes. According to Dr. Pusztai, tomatoes don't even contain this agent. Other possible reasons cited for these lesions were restriction in the rats' diet, but this is discredited by the fact that the rats were fed freely and ate as much as they wanted. Another named culprit was animal restraint, but the rats were not restrained.

Finally, Dr. Pusztai came upon an endnote in the Flavr Savr research documents that had not been addressed: He found that seven of the twenty rats fed the troublesome tomato line had died within two weeks. The death of these rats had been dismissed as a husbandry error, with scientists deciding to blame the feeding method rather than the food for the lesion. It was said that an error in inserting the feeding tubes had caused the rats to be injured by "accidental administration of test material into the lung instead of the stomach." But this explanation didn't address how that would cause *stomach* lesions and tumors; logic says the error would have injured the lung instead. The FDA scientists' own argument disproved their point.

Likewise, if it were true that the injuries were a result of the feeding procedure, then the number of lesions that manifested would have been more consistent between the two varying batches of test subjects and the different lines of tomatoes. Instead, the casualties were concentrated in just the one type of tomato. (Remember, these two types of tomatoes were created using identical materials, tools, and procedures.)

The doctor pointed this out, stating that certainly some of the rats that ate from the other tomato line would have died if the feeding method were the culprit. Again, this wasn't the case. With no additional explanation documented, a further shadow was cast by his investigation when he realized these lab rats were simply replaced with new ones, and the whole incident seemed to have been swept under the rug. The doctor noted that lab rats are not supposed to be replaced with new, living ones when they die during experimentation. Due diligence suggests that the death should be investigated, and the experiment should continue with the remaining live subjects. Introducing new rats could compromise the entire outcome of the experimentation. Additionally, postmortem analysis should be part of the procedure, especially when the goal is to determine whether a food or drug is "safe" for human consumption.

Of the stomach lesions, Dr. Pusztai, stated that equivalent injury to a human could have the potential to "lead to life-endangering hemorrhage, particularly in the elderly who used aspirin to prevent thrombosis."[17]

Some of the FDA scientists working on the study wrote memos saying that the rates of these lesions could not be discarded. Other scientists stated in their reports that these tomatoes fell below the FDA's standard of safety, despite that its regulations clearly require that these and any other GMOs be held to the same standard as other foods being approved.

The terminal lesions experienced by the lab rats were deemed by FDA authorities as "incidental," and they decided these issues had nothing to do with the tomatoes. Some FDA scientists were doubtful, claiming that the ambiguity around this study was still too much, but they were within the lower ranks of authority and were outnumbered; their concerns were disregarded.

In review, we started this look into the Flavr Savr tomatoes with two lines, or types, of tomatoes whose *only* variations were a result of the uniqueness that is unavoidable during the gene-insertion process. Out of one line, no rats died. Out of the other line, seven out of the twenty rats developed bleeding stomach lesions and died. This is a mortality rate of nearly 50 percent. If scientists were trying to advocate for making this tomato appear safe, one would imagine that there would have been a thorough investigation attempting to prove that feeding methods or lung damage were the concrete causes of death for these rats. This would have disavowed all doubt about the safety of the tomato.

Instead, concerns were left unaddressed and ambiguous evidence dismissed; later, some of the scientists involved even tried to say that no rats had died.[18] However, official reports documenting the process referred to "necroscopy data," which indicates a study performed on a dead body, not dead cells.

In addition to all of this, in trying to explain the deaths, some scientists' defense became that tomatoes, when eaten in excess, can kill rats. That leads one to wonder why tomatoes had been tested on rats in the first place. On top of everything else, that still doesn't answer the recurring question: Why did nearly half of one group of rats die, while there were no casualties from the other line?

At this point, one would wish that the FDA had exercised more caution in the approval process. One would have hoped for a longer period of testing, especially in light of the percentage of rats that showed up with complications. Further concern about the research on the Flavr Savr tomato included the fact that the rats used varied in weight, meaning that there wasn't a level playing field for gauging the animals' responses to the tomato in the first place.

With the FDA encouraged to promote public trust in biotechnology, the goal in approving the Flavr Savr tomato for sale to the public was surely to open the market to GMO foods. Investigations were essentially skimmed over, and concerns voiced by opposing scientists were ignored by the FDA officials in authority, who ultimately had the final say in whether this tomato was approved.

This was the beginning of a radical change in the food-supplying history of the world. The product was put on the market with very little research, which opened the door to more products of its kind. Unfortunately, no after-market research was conducted on the people consuming these products.

You might be thinking, "Why go into all of this history on a product that isn't even on the market anymore? This all happened during the '90s; surely food technology has come a long way since then! If this tomato isn't being sold to the public now, why should we care?"

We care because this case proves that since the introduction of GMO foods into our supermarkets, we've had no confirmation that these foods are safe. On the contrary, study results have been ambiguous at best, and shady and conspiratorial at worst.

This case shows that the first GMO experiment ever resulted in nearly 50 percent casualties for the lab rats that ate these products, and even indicates that since the introduction of GMO foods, the FDA and other powers that be have been disregarding risks to public health. For the sake of time and space limitations, we won't go through the history of all the GMO foods available, nor will we outline the investigations into each case, although concerns and results are similar. This example should suffice to show that since the beginning, "they" have not been looking out for our best interest, and GMOs are *abundantly available* in thousands of the foods we eat every day. There has been an underlying agenda from the onset of the GMO movement, with a supreme goal of getting GMOs on the market and into our bodies. Furthermore, when this movement is met with resistance, the concerns voiced are condescendingly deemed as "holding no scientific merit." Worse, scientists and others who try to voice concerns, like Dr. Pusztai, are ostracized, suspended, or otherwise silenced.

Adding to the GMO Threat

Another reason GMO foods are a threat is that they aren't labeled or monitored—and can even infect and contaminate our pure food sources. This means the potential for harm cannot be traced or measured. Additionally, when something new is introduced and no science to back it exists yet, the side effects can't be speculated upon. For example, if a person were on a prescription drug and side effects were to manifest, it would then be reasonable to research the medication that person had taken to pinpoint the cause of the side effects. With GMO foods, there is no such qualifying information yet: Our bodies are digesting food that nature never intended for us to take in, and the room for ambiguity as to the root of the symptoms is untraceably vast.

Taking in a GMO food places us at risk; adding this to the fact that many foods are processed and contain ingredients that are toxic means that our bodies are under a double attack. Many of these details will be highlighted in a later chapter, wherein we will discuss specific ingredients and why they are toxic to the body or mind. But to appreciate the drastic level at which these ingredients are affecting our psychology, physiology, and digestive systems, it is necessary to define excitotoxins and the blood-brain barrier. In the next chapter, we will discuss how the impact of these ingredients reaches farther than most people know.

4

Alarming Connections Beneath the Surface

The Blood-Brain Barrier

Between 1880 and 1913, scientists Paul Ehrlich and Edwin Goldman experimented on animals by injecting blue dye into their bloodstreams. When all the tissues of the body except the brain and spinal cord turned blue, the scientists theorized that something was isolating the brain from elements the rest of the body was exposed to. Another scientist, M. Lewandowsky, called this the "blood-brain barrier." Through their experimentation, these scientists determined that neurotoxic agents only affected brain function when they were directly injected to the brain. When these components were administered into the vascular system, the brain showed no reaction. It took the better part of one hundred years—seventy, to be exact—for two other scientists, T. S. Reese and M. J. Karnovsky, to pinpoint the location of the barrier, which they determined was the capillary endothelial cells within the brain. The endothelial cells and the brain capillaries, according to Neuroscience Online, "consists of a complex cellular system of a highly specialized basal membrane, a large number of pericytes embedded in the basal membrane and astrocytic end feet."[19] The endothelial cells of the brain are different from those found in other organs. The ones in the brain are connected, almost woven, in a tremendously tight fashion that keeps paracellular molecular movement from occurring, and they have no transendothelial pathways or intracellular vesicles. In a nutshell, it is a tightly woven barrier that only allows fat-soluble molecules, small molecules, and some gases into the brain. Larger molecules (such as glucose) have to pass through using a transporter protein, which essentially serves as the brain's way of filtering which molecules are allowed in and which must be blocked. This creates a type of "border" that keeps the blood in the brain chemistry separated and protected from occurrences within the rest of the body.

The blood-brain barrier is a safety system within the body that keeps foreign substances that are in the bloodstream out of the brain. For example, it blocks the ability of hormones and neurotransmitters from being able to cross over from the bloodstream into the brain, except through certain predesignated "doorways." This helps to keep the brain at a consistent level. When the blood-brain barrier is weakened, substances that should not be able to cross from the bloodstream into the brain are allowed through.

Some things that can weaken the blood-brain barrier are high blood pressure; any type of birth defect that keeps the blood-brain barrier from being fully developed at birth; hyperosmolility (this occurs when high levels of certain substances exist in the blood); microwaves or radiation; certain types of infection; or brain injury. The purpose of the blood-brain barrier is to protect the brain tissue from the variations that the rest of the body endures with the highs and lows of sugars, hormones, chemicals, agents, toxins, or anything else found in the rest of the body. As fluctuation within the body occurs around times of exercise, meals, illness, or even stress, the endothelial cells that form the blood-brain barrier are the gatekeepers of what is allowed into the brain.

Essential amino acids (coming from the blood because the brain cannot synthesize them) help move glucose into the brain. Metabolic processes performed in the brain capillary endothelial cells regulate the transference, or carrying, of neurotransmitters into the brain.

Circum-ventricular organs are specific locations in the brain that do not have a blood-brain barrier in place. These are the "doorways" within the barrier. This is where the hormone regulation between the blood and the brain takes place. Some examples are the pituitary gland, median eminence, pre-optic recess, the pineal gland, and the endothelium of choroid plexus. In these areas, the "weaving or knitting" of the endothelial cells is looser, allowing the molecular exchange.

Perhaps you have known of somebody who was abusing a substance and ended up vomiting as a result. When the body's toxin levels get so high that the blood-brain barrier is compromised, the circumventricular organ called the area postrema kicks in, causing the body to basically "evict" the toxic substance so that the level can be restored to a more manageable level, allowing the blood-brain barrier to continue protecting the brain from the toxic substance.

The blood-brain barrier is so effective that some drugs are unable to cross it. Scientists, experimenting with new drugs promised to treat diseases like Alzheimer's, find in their studies that some drugs have to be connected to a molecule or transporter protein to enter the brain's chemistry.

So why are we talking about the blood-brain barrier? Why is it so important?

Anytime something crosses the blood-brain barrier that is not supposed to enter the brain, it has a huge impact on our brain chemistry. Consider, for example the effect that certain diseases have on the blood-brain barrier. Meningococcal disease is particularly dangerous, because its bacteria binds to the endothelial wall, which results in small openings in this tightly woven barrier. This allows bacteria, toxins, and other compromising elements into the brain, which can lead to infections of the brain tissue, giving way for inflammation or even death. There are also other elements such as those mentioned earlier that affect the blood-brain barrier; this is only one example.

But there is more to consider than the effects of actual disease on the blood-brain barrier. Many of the ingredients *legally added to our food with FDA approval* cross the blood-brain barrier. Because so many of the foods we eat involve an excess of hormones, sugar, excitotoxins, and other chemicals that can cross this barrier, what we are eating doesn't only affect our bodies, but crosses this sovereignly placed barrier guarding our brain and having effects there as well. We're not simply eating foods that cause us to gain weight or munching on things that tinker with our blood sugar or blood pressure; we are changing our brain's chemistry.

We'll talk more about the spiritual application to this in the last part of the book, but for now, consider this: When you're eating food that is upsetting your brain's chemistry, over time, it has a long-term effect on *how you think*. Not only are we taking in ingredients that affect the physical aspect of how our bodies function, but these elements trigger emotional and biological reactions in our brains to the foods we are eating!

Excitotoxins

Now that you understand the basic concept of the blood-brain barrier, it is necessary to explain what an excitotoxin is, since the danger presented by your food means requiring an understanding of these two elements and how they go hand in hand. If you've never heard the word before, you may think that it has a villainously fictional ring to it, as if it were some sort of mad-scientist weaponry taken from an old-school comic book. However, the most nefarious villain in such cartoonish works of fiction could not have come up with a chemical warfare as potent and yet as capable of flying under the radar as your friendly local excitotoxin.

Excitotoxins are an element found in flavor enhancers. They are dangerous because they cross the blood-brain barrier. They are nonessential amino acids that stimulate the taste receptors or taste buds into believing the food has more flavor than it actually does.

Do you remember in your early adulthood, when you got your first credit card? Weren't you excited? You could have anything you wanted even if you didn't have the money! Maybe you bought some tires, or a tube of lipstick, or a cool new leather coat. Do you remember how you felt at the end of the month when your statement showed up? Perhaps you were one of those people who did well in the willpower department and kept the balance low. Or, maybe you were like so many others your age who learned this lesson the hard way, and whose gut sank immediately at seeing the accumulated balance. If you were in the latter group, then you probably had made a little purchase here, a little purchase there… and with each transaction, you forgot about the previous day's charges and the charges you had made even the day before that. Maybe you expected a bill of $150 or $200, only to learn at the end of the month that you had actually charged $600? It's a trap many fall into, and it's even easier to do this with food that has excitotoxins. A little bite here, a nibble there, and before you realize it, you've eaten more excitotoxins than you can account for.

Extremely alarming about excitotoxins is not only the fact that they cross the blood-brain barrier, but also that they trigger a neurological transmitter reaction in the brain that overstimulates the senses. This reaction within the brain is similar to a drug-induced high. As suggested by the name, these toxins "excite" the brain. After ingestion, the neurons within the brain began to fire erratically without cause. Several hours after those neurons fire, they die. They do not come back. Repeat: The brain does not renew them. *This damage cannot be undone.* Additional cell death occurs because of the elevated levels of free radicals and lipid peroxidation that result from the intake of excitotoxins. In lab animals, the increased levels of these free radicals and lipid peroxidation products are endured within the body for a period equivalent to decades for humans. Even more alarming than anything we've discussed yet is the fact that these chemicals not only cross the blood-brain barrier in a pregnant mother, but can actually cross the placental barrier as well, damaging the brain of the fetus. Of this connection, Dr. Edward Brown stated:

> When we eat foods laced with MSG or diet drinks sweetened with NutraSweet, the body is flooded with these excitatory neurotransmitter substances, to a level 5–20 times greater than normally present within the blood. This neurotransmitter excess can cause repetitive firing of neurons, and when this continues without rest, neurons can eventually fatigue and die. This is the origin of the term excitotoxin—the neurons are literally worked to death…. There is growing evidence that these artificial food additives accelerate neurodegeneration in the individuals with a genetic predisposition to condition such as Parkinson's disease, Alzheimer's dementia, and amyotrophic lateral sclerosis (ALS). Because these substances readily pass the placental barrier from mother to fetus, there is also speculation that MSG and NutraSweet have contributed toward the dramatic increase in attention deficit hyperactivity disorder (ADHD).[20]

Over time, the "high" of this experience literally addicts people to food and dulls their brain's ability to function, increasing vulnerability to mental illness. The population is riddled with people who, unwittingly, are either addicted to food or suffering mentally (or both) because of excitotoxins. They don't realize the price they're paying for the taste they're experiencing is much higher than they know. As stated, excitotoxins cross the blood-brain barrier and stimulate the brain. Over time, their effect "stacks up" in the brain, leading to much more serious consequences. Some of the long-term prices to be paid for this are Lou

Gehrig's Disease, Alzheimer's, and other forms of disease that contribute to dementia.

In the meantime, we're also feeding our children these stimulants. The average "fruit" snacks are loaded with excitotoxins. The impact of excitotoxins is far more extensive than that of the food dyes, preservatives, and multiple sugars that are in these products. Because the body responds to excitotoxins nearly immediately, kids become hyperactive and are then diagnosed with behavioral disorders (more on this later).

Excitotoxins, because they are a stimulant, have been linked to many problems ranging from hormonal disorders to violent behaviors. They cause brain-cell death, sexual development and fertility problems, and have been named as directly contributing to mental illness. Excitotoxins have also been linked to neurological side effects, headaches, sleep disorders, seizures, epilepsy, and paralysis. Excitotoxins such as cysteine (made from human hair and poultry feathers!) have been associated with neurodegenerative damage—wherein is the link to Parkinson's, Alzheimer's, and Lou Gehrig's disease. Other linked issues are amyotrophic lateral sclerosis, strokes, heart attack, heart disease, brain injury, brain tumors, neurological Lyme disease, encephalitis, schizophrenia, migraines, and seizures. A large majority of the complications caused by excitotoxins are irreversible.

Sadly, these brain-damaging toxins are even found in some of our "health foods," with the endorsement of the FDA! Understand—these have absolutely no health value and no nutritional value whatsoever. They are nothing more than a mere chemical added to our food to make it "taste better." Excitotoxins hide out in our food under other names such as MSG or aspartame, although there are many others.

Glutamate is an excitotoxin that often appears on the health foods lists, posing as a friend. Because the body uses glutamate as one of the main neurotransmitters of the brain, some people have fallen for the lie that it's safe to eat, but it isn't. It's true that a very small amount of glutamate *does* play a role in our cellular function, but its role is limited, and the brain generates it *as needed*. At the time that the brain *needs* this substance, it generates the precise amount it requires. For the brain to be flooded with this substance when it is not needed is detrimental to the brain's signaling system, throwing it off base. Additionally, when the brain does produce glutamate, it does so in tiny amounts. When glutamate is consumed in food, it is at a much higher concentration than the brain would generate on its own, overloading the signal center of the brain.

The worst part about this is that scientists have been telling about the dangers of excitotoxins since the 1950s. Yes, that's right—we are approaching nearly seventy years of unheeded warnings regarding these extremely dangerous chemicals!

Serious concern about excitotoxins date as far back as 1957, when researchers attempted to repair the diseased retina of a lab rat using glutamate.[21] Instead, they found that not only did the glutamate fail to perform as expected, but it caused the retinal cells to be altogether destroyed. Later, further investigation showed that the entire brain was compromised by the use of glutamate. The hypothalamus, a tiny organ in the brain that plays a key role in hormonal function, can be destroyed by an excessive intake of MSG (of which Americans have consumed 282,000 metric tons since the 1980s[22]) or other excitotoxins. In 1981, some doctors within the FDA did not support the approval of aspartame, because mice experimented on using the substance developed brain tumors. Former FDA toxicologist Dr. Adrian Gross even testified before the US Senate, saying, "It is clear beyond any shadow of a doubt that aspartame has caused cancer in laboratory animals."[23] Some experts argue that excitotoxins are not the direct cause of neurological diseases, but even they are unable to deny that research consistently proves a direct link between excitotoxins and the susceptibility to the previously mentioned diseases. So what does this mean for us? Food companies are (legally) adding to our groceries chemicals that literally "mess with our head." They overstimulate taste receptors, leading us to crave food when we do not need to eat. Excitotoxins create the impression within our brain that we are hungry when we are not. On top of this, it interrupts brain function, compromises our general health, and causes cell death within the brain that leads to dementia-related illness in the elderly and behavioral disorders in children. Why does the FDA allow this to continue? That is the million-dollar question. If the FDA were looking out for the general health of the public, these chemicals would be illegal.

Before you assume that you are free from the risk presented by these excitotoxins because you're eating natural food, beware. Unfortunately, MSG is only one type of excitotoxin, and it hides under at least thirty different names. Upwards of seventy types of excitotoxins are added to our food these days. Just the simple word "spice" can be a signal word for MSG.

If you're feeling overwhelmed by learning all of this, you are not alone.

This is where consumer vigilance must play a role. Even listed label ingredients like "natural flavoring" can contain excitotoxins, so we must watch labels and investigate what products actually contain. Calling the phone number on the label and asking for elaboration on an ingredient may be necessary. Eventually, you will establish lists of brands that you do and do not trust. Refuse to buy anything with flavor enhancers or other excitotoxins. Carefully screening brands and learning which ones you can trust will get easier with practice. When in doubt, a good rule of thumb is what my mom taught us when we worked in food service: *When in doubt, don't.* The variety of foods on your menu may narrow for a while, but you will eventually replace them with safer options. How to simplify your menu and eat more homemade foods will be covered later in this book.

If the idea of removing excitotoxins from your diet seems daunting, take heart. Most of the time, these ingredients are found in processed food. So, if you simply decide to remove processed food from your diet, you're likely to eliminate many of these dangerous chemicals from your diet. It will not be easy; even restaurants that boast "no MSG" on signs in their windows are likely buying products that are loaded with the substance. Make inquiries into what, exactly, is being served at restaurants that you frequent. Make up your mind to make small improvements (more on this later) all the time, and take each eliminated or embraced product as one small victory. Remember, each time you purchase something or do not purchase something, you are essentially voting with your money. If the excitotoxin market is driven by consumer demand, then we can make a difference by demanding no excitotoxins in our food.

More Addicting Than Cocaine...

An ingredient that needs to be addressed as more than just marginally dangerous is sugar, when it is ingested in excess. There is a safe threshold of sugar, but most Americans bypass this amount before they even finish breakfast. According to the American Heart Association, the maximum amount of added sugar you should eat in a day is: for men, 37.5 grams, and for women, 25 grams.[24] To put perspective on this, one can of Coke contains 33 grams, an average coffee shop's extra-large white chocolate mocha with whipped cream has almost 74 grams,[25] and the average blueberry muffin runs between 37–40 grams of sugar. This means that *any sugar* the average person ingests after breakfast is too much. To give you further perspective, 1 gram of sugar burns the equivalent of 4 calories, and an hour spent on a treadmill for the average adult will burn roughly 300 calories. It is then an approximate average that one hour on a treadmill will burn 75 grams of sugar.

In 2002, the World Health Organization, along with the Food and Agricultural Organization of the United Nations, held a consultation on diet, nutrition, and the prevention of chronic illness. The resulting report, the *Technical Report Series No. 916 (TRS 916)*, outlined details on dietary and physical activity elements contributing to chronic illness, including diabetes and obesity. This report recommended that people limit their daily intake of sugar to 10 percent of their overall calories. Countries exporting sugar and producers of sugar immediately answered this recommendation with concerns of their own: This kind of consumer restraint could cause a crash for the sugar-based industry. Sales lost could be disastrous, since sugar is one of the largest food commodities in the world. The debate became one of nutrition and health versus industry and profits. Tommy Thompson, the secretary of Health and Human Services at that time, flew to Geneva to relay the message that the US government would withhold $406 million in funding, should the report be published.[26]

While this debate spurred constructive action within many countries of the world, the largest effect the American consumer might see is that the percentage of daily recommended allowance, found on the nutrition label of our food products, is no longer displayed to the right of sugar. The US Institute of Medicine still maintains that 25 percent of daily caloric intake can safely come from added sugar.[27]

Princeton University Professor Bart Hoebel recently presented evidence gathered by the Princeton University Department of Psychology and the Princeton Neuroscience Institute showing that sugar is as addictive as other drugs such as cocaine, heroin, or morphine. Rats addicted to sugar showed signs of craving, relapse, withdrawal, and changes within the brain, confirming addiction.[28]

> Hoebel has shown that rats eating large amounts of sugar when hungry, a phenomenon he described as sugar-binging, undergo neurochemical changes in the brain that appear to mimic those produced by substances of abuse, including cocaine morphine and nicotine. Sugar induces behavioral changes, too. "In certain models, sugar–binging causes long-lasting effects in the brain and increases the inclination to take other drugs of abuse, such as alcohol," Hoebel said....

Hungry rats that binge on sugar provoke a surge of dopamine in their brains. After a month, the structure of the brains of these rats adapts to increased dopamine levels, showing fewer of a certain type of dopamine receptor than they used to have and more opioid receptors. These dopamine and opioid systems are involved in motivation and reward, systems that control wanting and liking something. Similar changes also are seen in the brains of rats on cocaine and heroin.[29]

Director of the Comprehensive Weight Control Center at New York-Presbyterian Hospital/Weill Cornell Medical Center, Dr. Louis Aronne, said of people experiencing sugar addiction, "These people get strong urges to consume sweets, and these cravings border on addiction. When they eat sugar, just like when someone ingests cocaine, some people get that feeling of well-being, a rush that makes them feel good for a period of time. When the sweets are taken away, the people just don't feel right."[30]

Rats in the withdrawal state from sugar experienced symptoms similar to those of an addict deprived of heroin, cocaine, morphine, or other drugs. They isolated themselves in a small part of their cage, their teeth chattered, they remained withdrawn, they displayed signs of anxiety, they quivered, and they showed disinterest in things they would normally be curious about.

Dr. Serge Ahmed of the University of Bordeaux in France, who believes that sugar is actually *more* addictive than cocaine, said, "When society finally discovers that refined sugar is just another white powder, along with pure cocaine, it will change its mind and attitude toward refined food addiction."[31]

Sugar, consumed in excess (even "good, old-fashioned white sugar"), is completely toxic and detrimental to the system. In the documentary *Fed Up*, Dr. Robert Lustig, professor of pediatrics at the University of California, San Francisco, said this:

Sugar is poison. It is a chronic—not acute—chronic, dose-dependent—depends on how much you eat, because there is a safe threshold—hepato, "liver" toxin. The metabolic diseases that are associated with obesity: the diabetes, heart disease, the lipid problems, the strokes, the cancer.... Those diseases are being driven by sugar.[32]

Because excessive sugar causes an overload of insulin that then interferes with the signal that we are full, the brain believes the body to be starving, even though the body is overloaded. This results in feelings of sluggishness, fatigue, and of course, hunger, which causes us to eat more, further feeding obesity.

If sugar were only in the places that we were looking for it, we would know to simply ease off the desserts to curb our sugar intake. But sugar hides under so many names and in so many unexpected products—think sports drinks, fruit products, crackers, even salad dressings—it is nearly impossible to avoid without hypervigilance.

Sugar from fruit is balanced with an amount of fiber that cancels out the negative effects of the sugar. Changing to artificial sugar is not an answer, because many artificial sweeteners are excitotoxins that, beyond the risks already outlined earlier in this chapter, trigger hormonal effects that cause the body to produce more insulin. This makes us crave more sugar. As stated before, most of us have exceeded the daily allowance of sugar before we even finishing breakfast, meaning that we will never burn off all the sugar we consume. In addition to this, these sugar-induced calories that convert into energy so rapidly cause the body to stop burning fat, which results in stubborn, hard-to-lose belly fat. (Remember, I mentioned earlier that, despite my weight loss, I couldn't lose the belly fat.)

Studies showing that sugar is as addictive as cocaine or heroin confirm that food addiction is not a myth. It's a fact. When added to the high caused by excitotoxins, the biological addiction many have to food is one that could be as hard to shake as any other addiction.

For research purposes, I am holding a 32-ounce sport drink. I will not mention the brand of this "thirst aid," but you probably know the one. The label shows a serving size to be 8 fluid ounces. Because it is a 32-ounce bottle, it is reasonable to assume that the consumer is expected to drink the entire bottle. On the nutrition label, the first ingredient listed is water. That's followed immediately by sucrose, then glucose-fructose syrup. The amount of sugar in one serving is listed at 14 grams. Because the manufacturer has divided the bottle into four servings, the ingredient quantities on the label are divided by four as well. As a result, the consumer is unknowingly (unless they read the label carefully) consuming four times the sugar reported on the label. If I were to drink this entire bottle of sports drink, I would be consuming 56 grams of sugars. This is only one way we must be vigilant about the manufacturers' tendencies to hide ingredients in plain sight. In a later chapter, we will discuss how to carefully read labels to avoid being caught in these traps of overconsumption.

Follow the Money

It can be hard to know what is true and what is false with all the media messages surrounding food-related issues, but it is correct what they say: The shortest distance between two points is a straight line. And that line is usually the money.

You may recall several years ago, when television commercials aired claiming that high-fructose corn syrup was "just sugar." These commercials, sponsored by the Corn Refiners Association, claimed that high-fructose corn syrup was just as safe as any regular sugar. But who were the major financial backers behind this campaign?

Six studies were conducted to render the consumer's image of high-fructose corn syrup to be as safe as regular sugar. Of the six, three were backed by companies that stood to gain financially from the statement that high-fructose corn syrup would be as safe as regular sugar. One was Pepsi, one was the American Beverage Association, and one was a Washington DC group funded by food, chemical, and drug companies.[33]

Of this scenario and others similar, Dr. Joseph Mercola said:

It's a widely known fact that when a study is sponsored by a company with financial interests in the outcome, the results rarely do anything but support the industry that funded the study.… In fact, CBS mentions a study by Children's Hospital Boston that found when studies were sponsored exclusively by food or drinks companies, the results were 4 to 8 times more likely to be favorable to the sponsoring company. So when the Corn Refiners Association claims that their deceptive $20–30 million ad campaign promoting corn syrup is "based on nutritional research," now you know just what type of biased research they are using.[34]

The sugar industry, not to be slighted or shortchanged, responded to this campaign by suing the Corn Refiners Association, claiming (in this case truthfully) that the commercials were both "inaccurate and misleading to consumers."[35] But were sugar industry advocates *really* looking out for the consumer? Of course not! They were using their own counterattack against this campaign to retrieve sales being diverted from sugar commerce and into the corn industry.

However, in a situation such as this, a campaign of finger-pointing never brings about as much success as a campaign "for the benefit of the people," so that is *precisely* the angle the sugar industry took. It rallied behind the façade of showing concern for "the health of the consumer." Of course, we all know what the motivation was. Within big business, we must watch for the repeated tactic of side-swiping the other guy under the heading of "consumer health" while the consumers are being manipulated and our health is being compromised for the gain of his dollar.

This was a rare occasion of an agenda behind an ad campaign being exposed. (Many times, their guises are successful and their products are embraced by a trusting population.) During the aftermath, soft-drink companies that had previously helped fund this fraudulent campaign showed their true colors by flipping sides, proudly advertising slogans like "Made with Real Sugar!" on their products.

The point in bringing this issue up: Any campaign that reassures consumers that its synthetic material is safe to ingest is likely funded by an agency with an interest in its results, and will likely be disproven over time. And even when truth is "exposed," it could be done so under a hidden agenda as well, leaving loyal backers to change their position in pursuit of the almighty dollar. Buyer beware.

Another example of this type of strategy can be seen when we examine Michelle Obama's "Let's Move" campaign. When the First Lady announced on February 9, 2010, that she would be launching a campaign against childhood obesity, many people rallied to her support, regardless of which side of the presidential election they had been on. People across the states supported the movement. It seemed that schools everywhere prepared for the lunch-program overhaul inevitably coming. At the start, one of the goals was to get food manufacturers to "pursue their calorie reduction goals by growing and introducing lower-calorie options; changing product recipes where possible to lower the calorie content of current products; or reducing portion sizes of existing single-serve products."[36] Early on, the campaign was pushed with talk of fresh vegetables, obesity awareness, and exercise among children in schools. In May of the same year, Michelle Obama announced that the Partnership for a Healthier America had signed an agreement with the Healthy Weight Commitment Foundation, agreeing that 1.5 trillion product calories would be reduced from food marketed to children, particularly in schools. This ultimately resulted in smaller portion sizes of the same types of food. Schools began to offer more fresh veggies and fruit, but unfortunately, many kids rejected the new healthier foods being offered.

School cafeteria staff ran into the additional obstacle of labeling criteria. Paperwork that became necessary to qualify for the mandatory six cents per tray that eventually resulted from this movement required that exact counts for carbs, proteins, sugars, etc. were documented in detail. This may seem like a good idea, and surely it's a step in the right direction, but it rendered a lot of homemade foods more difficult to qualify. Time efficiency and staffing issues in many schools caused the last few homemade recipes to be shelved in favor of a pizza slice or corn dog with a well-documented nutrition label. Debate began to take place over details that led astray from the heart of the matter. Resources were wasted on such debates as whether a slice of pizza had enough tomato paste to be considered a vegetable serving. The answer was eventually set at qualifying one slice of pizza as one-eighth of a cup of tomato. Eventually, the focus of the program shifted from the quality of food being served to kids at school to exercise. What changed?

Food conglomerates that stepped in "endorsing" the program were also given enough pull to distract from the core issues. What was presented as a movement for children's health became another channel through which industry was able to regulate and control what is being fed to our kids at school. To confirm what I am saying, note that the Healthy Weight Commitment Foundation is comprised of a board of directors and governors who hail from the following major food companies: PepsiCo, Nestlé, the Coca-Cola Company, General Mills, Inc., the Hershey Company, Grocery Manufacturers Association, Shearers Snacks, Hy-Vee, Inc., and Bumble Bee Seafoods. Since these are parent companies that own many of the large corporations that sell mass quantities of prefabricated foods to our schools, these entities had an interest in the jurisdiction that would come out of this program. In the end, much of the food served at schools remained the same, but it was reintroduced in smaller portion sizes and relabeled accordingly, just like the sport drink described previously.

On top of all of this, while overall calorie counts or sugar contents may *now read differently* on your child's cafeteria lunch tray, it doesn't change the fact that your children are eating the same excitotoxin-riddled, preservative-filled, artificially flavored and colored GMO food they were eating before. We never did get to the *core issue* for our children. To say that the "Let's Move" campaign did nothing beneficial would not be true. The campaign raised awareness and kick-started an attitude of proactivity about obesity among the kids within our schools. But unfortunately, when big money enters the scene, ambiguity and agenda began to cloud what might otherwise be progress.

The Financial Fallout

Circumstances surrounding the manufacturing of the food we eat are so convoluted that they leave consumers unsure of where the cycle begins and ends, and maybe even a little paranoid about which manufacturers can be trusted. It seems there are no clean lines around our food industry. Corporations subsidized by the government supply to larger food conglomerates. The same government subsidizing the agricultural industries that supply the food conglomerates is also responsible for regulating safety of products sold. This on its own should be considered a conflict of interests, but when we also consider that the government is also largely involved in our healthcare, that complicates everything. On one hand, it is propping up agricultural products sold to large conglomerates to be used as unsafe ingredients in fatty, cheap foods. On the other hand, they are charged with making sure the products being sold are safe. When they become additionally involved in our healthcare, we begin to wonder if it all is just part of one big monetary cycle, with the general population at the hub. Throw into the complicated mix the health insurance companies that are now investing in fast-food companies,[37] and it paints a devastatingly clear picture: The money we are saving on cheaper groceries is being spent on sustaining the illness that our cheaper food causes. This is a growing industry. Here are some staggering progressive statistics: Within two decades, over 95 percent of our American population will be overweight or obese, and within thirty years, we will reach a one-in-three ratio for cases of diabetes.[38] There is a lot to be gained by selling unhealthy food at a cheaper price when these agencies are all holding hands.

Dr. Robert Lustig, professor of pediatrics at the University of California in San Francisco, stated: "The financial aspects of this are staggering. [Seventy-five] percent of our healthcare dollar goes to the maintenance or treatment of chronic metabolic disease."[39]

Dr. Harvey Karp, assistant professor of pediatrics for the Keck School of Medicine at the University of Southern California, stated about the same issue: "If you think the national debt is a problem right now, wait till you see the tsunami of debt that's coming from the health care impact of obesity."[40]

This debt will be funneled through our tax system because of the hand the government now has in our healthcare as citizens. This is debt that our children will be saddled with because of our lack of vigilance over our own health. Much of the information shared in this book has been kept under wraps for fifty years. Just as the industries delayed action where tobacco was concerned, a similar filibuster is taking place within the realms of legislation and regulation between food conglomerates and our government. And, just like the situation with tobacco, by the time necessary action is taken, many lives will have been ruined or lost.

Handing Down the Problem

Another troubling fact that many people don't know is that our DNA can adapt to the dietary changes we implement in our own bodies. These changes can then be inherited by our children. Dr. Mercola made this alarming statement about the possibility that what we're eating will cause our children to suffer:

It's now well known that dietary changes can prompt epigenetic DNA changes that can be passed on to future generations. For instance, pregnant rats fed a fatty diet had daughters and granddaughters with a greater risk of breast cancer. It could be that we are just now starting to see these types of generational effects showing up in humans, caused by our grandparents' and parents' penchant for processed foods. If that's the case, then we have even more incentive to make drastic changes, and soon, because the disease trends we are now seeing are only going to get worse as much of the processed foods consumed today are *not even food based!* So who knows what kind of genetic mutations and malfunctions we are creating for our future generations when a MAJORITY of our diet consists of highly processed and artificial foods. As it stands, 90 percent of foods Americans purchase every year are processed foods![41]

Knowing that what we eat can change the physical traits we hand down to our children literally means that the health that's been granted to us is our responsibility to pay forward to our children. They deserve it, and they're counting on us for it. Once I knew that I had been contributing to my own health problems, even after I had been trying to make "better choices" with food while the answers were hidden in plain sight all the while, it bothered me. What really hurt, though, was remembering the times that I had "treated" my kids with sugary cereals or pizza. It broke my heart to think of the times they had earned some sort of reward, and I had given it to them in the form of something harmful. Further, I was helping create an association for them of "fun and reward" coming in the form of something toxic. It is important that we take care of our own bodies for the sake of our children and our grandchildren, yet unborn, just the same way we would adjust the way we are feeding the ones who have already been born.

5

The Rabbit Hole Is Deep, In Every Way

Big Pharma/Big Agri-Link

In a society that values the "quick fix" over a long-term solution, our health habits have become a casualty of our busy lifestyles. When we're sick, the typical medical standard is to treat our symptoms and dismiss the core problem until the symptoms become tenacious enough to keep surfacing. This superficial treatment of physical symptoms creates a climate within our bodies where a deeper problem can remain in hiding, escalating all the while. Besides the obvious fact that an undiagnosed medical problem can eventually become lethal when it is finally discovered, much of the medication we take regularly is as dangerous as, if not worse than, the food we're eating. This becomes a cycle that propels itself: We eat food that is not healthy, we take medicine to mask the symptoms, and the medicine's side effects make us sick. That creates the need for another medication, which then triggers other, new side effects. The only way to break this cycle is to stay healthy in the first place. But how do we stay ahead of all this when it seems like the system works against us? And what or who is at the center of this cycle? Are we trapped in a set of circumstances that is the byproduct of a series of unfortunate events, or is a more nefarious force orchestrating this from the inside out?

It is obvious that eating the wrong foods, or too much food, makes us sick. We will talk more about that in upcoming pages. But for now, let's examine a connection between our big factory farms, the pharmaceutical industry, and the food conglomerates. *Grist* author Amelia Urry sums it up best:

> Since 1995, 75 percent of federal subsidies have gone to 10 percent of farms, the same consolidated group of commodity crop growers who will continue to eat up a disproportionate share of the subsidy pie under the new system, too.
>
> These payments fund a massive industrialized food system that takes its toll on our land and water, while our diets are full of all that extra corn, from our corn-fed burgers to our Halloween candy—and so are our cars.
>
> Now picture the world we could live in if we subsidized the food that actually feeds people, and feeds local economies all the while. Just think! We could save money on healthcare and spend it paying for things we actually want, like well-managed land, cleaner water, a diversified localized economy, and some fresh, organic sweet corn.[42]

It is no secret that a large percentage of subsidized farming is made up of corn agriculture. Granted, not all corn farmed under subsidies ends up on our grocery shelves, and not every aspect of agricultural subsidization is bad. But consider how many artificial sweeteners are made of corn. And the industry has yet to produce a healthy synthetic sweetener option. What we have then is our tax dollars at work subsidizing the agriculture that's behind the manufacturing of products that are killing us.

Beyond this, the variety of corn-based sweeteners creates the next level of deception for the consumer. For example, high-fructose corn syrup is the most commonly known of the sweeteners, but others include glucose syrup, dextrose, maltodextrin, erythritol, and many others. As I write this, I am holding a package of children's fruit-flavored snacks featuring a well-loved, popular cartoon character. The front label boasts such selling points as: "Only 80 calories per serving," "Now with NO artificial flavors," and "NO calories from artificial sources."

The ingredients label follows:

Corn syrup, sugar, modified corn starch, pear juice concentrate, apple juice concentrate. Contains 2% or less of: citric acid, fruit pectin, sodium citrate, malic acid, dextrose, color (vegetable juice, fruit juice, spirulina extract and turmeric extract), potassium citrate, vitamin C (ascorbic acid), sunflower oil, natural flavor, and carnauba wax.

Bear in mind that this product is advertised as a kids' snack and is not marketed as a candy, and review the ingredients again. The following are synthetic, commonly used ingredients made from corn: corn syrup, modified corn starch, and dextrose. In addition, listings such as "concentrate juice," "vegetable juice," and "natural flavor" leaves the product open for additional, unlabeled ingredients to be smuggled into this snack. In trying to find out what is in such products, we find the labeling ambiguous at best.

Understanding that most of these ingredients are stated to comprise less than 2 percent of the product, 98 percent of the product is therefore made up of the first five ingredients. This tells us the snack is mainly comprised of sugar and corn. Some may argue on behalf of nutrition because of the fruit juices included, but that position doesn't hold water. When fruit juice is made, the fruit is pressed and fibers are removed while the fluids are retained, creating juice. Essentially, this means that the "sugar water" within the fruit is being separated from the rest of its nutrients. While this *is* a sugar from fruit, it still is not a healthy form of sugar for the body to ingest, because it has been stripped from its necessary co-ingredients, which play key a role in how the body processes sugar from fruit. (This is the essence of why so many debate whether fruit juice is healthy.) So including juice, even at its most nutritious, doesn't guarantee that the product is healthy or has any nutritional value. On top of this, without a guarantee that artificial sweeteners are not included in this concentrate juice, there's no certainty that further additional synthetic sweeteners, even excitotoxins, haven't been added.

This collection of information is meant to show that, as stated before, tax dollars subsidize the corn industry, which is responsible for myriad synthetic ingredients that are toxic or lack nutritional value. Those are then mislabeled and packaged in a way that "appears harmless" (with FDA approval). We then purchase these products and feed them to our children. Nearly 75 percent of modern-day Americans fall into the obese category.[43] In contrast to the subsidies doled out to industries like corn, sugar, and soy, to name a few, there is little subsidization offered to farmers of fresh fruits and vegetables. Wouldn't it be much better if we could take a significant percentage of the currently disbursed subsidy money and channel it into agriculture that raises organic fruits and vegetables?

It may seem like I am picking on the corn industry. I am using it only as an example. Many other subsidized agricultural products (soy, for example) are responsible for dangerous synthetic products as well. My goal is not to pick on any one industry; it is to point out the vicious, self-perpetuating cycle that does a disservice to the citizens whose back-breaking labor is at the hub, earning the money that pays the tax dollars that subsidize our own demise.

Begin at Home

The abundance of convenient, fatty, sugary foods available coupled with the continuing economic squeeze many families are enduring mean that consumers are easily lured into a trap wherein healthy foods are replaced with cheaper junk food at the price of health instead of the wallet. School lunches, despite Michelle Obama's overhaul, still in large part feature processed foods. In addition, food insecurity at home sabotages progress made within the realms of public food service endeavors such as school lunch programs. In an interview regarding children's responses to healthier options at lunch, one "lunch lady" at a local middle school said:

> You can't do anything about it if they don't know what healthy food is to begin with. We served pears and the kids thought they were deformed apples. We served deli-style sandwich wraps with alfalfa sprouts inside and the kids threw them away, thinking we had served them some sort of grass burrito. When we served the meatloaf, they thought it was "really gross looking chocolate cake!"

She went on to relate her frustration with how much healthy food was being thrown away. The work it takes to wash, prep, and cut produce requires extra staff and effort at a school kitchen, and cafeteria staff finds it demoralizing to watch the kids scoff at it and throw it away because they've never seen anything like it before. So, unfortunately, schools that are more diligent about offering fresh fruits and vegetables find that children whose appetites (or exposure) have not adapted to healthy food simply waste the nutritious food. Further, we can't forget that processed, fatty, sugary foods are biologically addictive, causing whole foods to lose the competition for our appetites. Efforts toward awareness are now placing emphasis on the individual to make better choices, and this is vital to bringing about change on a large scale. But in settings like our local schools, where children are in large part biologically addicted to processed food and lack the foresight and willpower to care about the long-term ramifications of processed food on their bodies, the people trying to make a change are outnumbered without support from home.

As long as markets that are subsidized continue to produce foods that are cheap, dangerous, and addictive, demand for these items likewise escalates. Healthy foods, which tend to be more expensive because they usually are not subsidized on an agricultural level, become lost in the mix and seem to lack the advantageous, "competitive edge" of the unhealthy food. As this happens, obesity, diabetes, and other chronic illnesses begin to thrive within the population. Manufacturers of these foods are also flourishing—as we see in their high volumes of sales. Industries such as these will not initiate a change that the people don't want; why would they? This is how the large food conglomerates make their millions. If people continue to purchase their convenience foods, these industries will go right along making them and selling them at high volumes, perpetuating the cycle that (as our interview with the school lunch cafeteria worker shows) begins at home. And as the general population becomes sicker, we become "feeder fish" for the next in line behind the food conglomerates to take our dollars: the pharmaceutical industry. I should mention that though it took a couple of months, my children's palates have adapted to s healthier diet, and now they *love* Alaskan salmon, bone-broth stews, sweet potatoes, and a plethora of other healthy foods that have become our go-to nutrition.

The Pharmaceutical Angle

Where does the pharmaceutical industry take us? Back to the FDA. According to Dr. David Graham, associate director for science and medicine in the Office of Drug Safety at FDA, every day that a new drug is awaiting approval represents a \$1–2 million loss for its manufacturing agency.[44] Because of this, the FDA is under intense pressure to get drugs approved quickly. In response, the Prescription Drug User Fee Act was passed in 1992, allowing drug companies to pay the FDA for speedy approval of their products. Sadly, the byproduct of this turn of events is that the agency that is supposed to keep us safe is actually being paid by those who want our money to approve medicines that may have dangerous side effects. This creates a conflict of interests: Under these circumstances, how can the FDA be objective and cautious, keeping human safety at top priority, without funding being compromised?

On this matter, Dr. David Graham said:

The FDA is not able to adequately protect the American public. It's more interested in protecting the interests of industry. It views industry as its client, and the client is someone whose interest you represent. Unfortunately, that is the way the FDA is currently structured. Within the Center for Drug Evaluation and Research about 80 percent of the resources are geared towards the approval of new drugs and 20 percent is for everything else. Drug safety is about five percent. The "gorilla in the living room" is new drugs and approval. Congress has not only created that structure, they have also worsened that structure through the PDUFA, the Prescription Drug User Fee Act, by which drug companies pay money to the FDA so they will review and approve its drug.

About the issue of drug safety, Dr. Graham added:

I'm really not at liberty to talk about things that pertain to my official duties at the FDA. I can talk in my private capacity, but I can't talk about material that would be confidential. What I can say is that there are a number of other scientists within the FDA who have also worked with drugs that they know are not safe, even though the FDA has approved or allowed them to remain on the market. They face some of the same difficulties that I do. The difference is that either the problem isn't as serious in terms of the numbers of people that were injured or that it's a fatal reaction—they're not willing to expose themselves to retaliation by the FDA—and retaliation would surely follow.

Dr. Graham has worked within the FDA to remove drugs that are not safe, and was even labeled a whistleblower before his Senate testimony in November 2004. Before his testimony, he admitted that he was essentially bullied in an effort to discourage him from testifying (the whole set of circumstances could merit its own chapter). Suffice it to say that within the FDA there are scientists who can attest to the fact that there is a conflict of interests that is compromising people's safety. Of the FDA, Graham said, "They know that they've disserved the American people. The FDA is responsible for 140,000 heart attacks and 60,000 dead Americans."[45]

Gwendolyn Leslie Olsen, a fifteen-year former sales rep within the pharmaceutical industry, outlines her experiences in that industry in her book, *Confessions of an RX Drug Pusher*. She outlines that in the FDA approval process, as few as two studies must show statistical effectiveness. According to Olsen, a drug can fail several times as long as it can manifest the correct results at least twice. On top of this, "less than 50% of the serious adverse reactions to a new drug are identified by the FDA before its release on the market."[46] Essentially, Olsen explains, because of financial influence and an endless list of drugs awaiting approval, products are rushed through the approval process without thorough testing. The post-marketing, drug-risk assessment conducted after the release of a new medication is abbreviated due to lack of staffing in this department, a scenario that Olsen calls "the largest Phase IV clinical trial population on the planet."[47] Even at this, the FDA estimates that, at most, 10 percent of negative side effects are reported. This means that as the populace embraces a new medication, expecting health and relief of symptoms, they are actually being experimented on by an agency that has taken funding for the approval of the medication, letting due diligence slip through the cracks.

Olsen maintains that most physicians she interacted with were well meaning, but they were given biased information about medications in an effort to see the pharmaceuticals prescribed in high volumes. Once out of medical school, educational information, seminars, or other available training was often funded by pharmaceutical companies, creating a further conflict of interests. In 2003, drug companies spent more than $1,500 per year on CME (continuing medical education) for each doctor in the United States.[48]

Olsen also outlined several types of manipulation the pharmaceutical industry uses against a trusting public to spike its own sales and line its pockets. Some came in the form of public service campaigns or announcements to "raise awareness" about various illnesses and disorders. In these campaigns, viewers are made to doubt their own quality of life, are pointed to a pharmaceutical solution, and are then encouraged to ask their doctor if the product is right for them. In microscopic fine print at the very bottom of the screen or pamphlet, downplayed side effects appear listed as an afterthought. Patients then ask their doctors about the matter out of curiosity born of this new "awareness." Because the doctor will have recently been introduced to the medication by his pharmaceutical rep, he will respond positively and quite possibly prescribe the product to the patient. By bypassing both the doctor and the need for symptoms and going straight to the patient, prompting their inquiry, the pharmaceutical industry gains high revenue selling meds to patients who may never have even thought to complain about their symptoms.

The worst part about Olsen's recollection as a pharmaceutical rep was her accounting of the manipulation of medical doctors. According to Olsen, a pharmaceutical representative is to befriend the doctor, to appear to be a professional comrade, and even to become a personal friend. She tells stories of buying meals in private rooms in restaurants, dropping lunch off at offices, delivering gift baskets and holiday gifts, and even sending singing telegrams to gain favorable status with these professionals. She reported that these efforts caused sales to spike so dramatically that her investments were always returned. Many states have introduced legislation that safeguards against these dramatic types of gift-giving, but it nevertheless indicates that the pharmaceutical industry is using every possible method of getting us on their medicine and keeping us on it.

While it is probably true that the FDA is spread too thin to adequately and objectively regulate pharmaceuticals as it should, it seems that there is still an ironic propensity toward taking control over more fields. Even today, as I was preparing to submit the manuscript of this book to the editor, a new article circulated the Internet, stating that the FDA was making plans to "crack down on homeopathic remedies."[49] In the article, the reasons cited were that the FDA allegedly had concerns about trusting people who spent their money on what they called "therapies that may bring little to no benefit in combating serious ailments."[50] But when putting this picture together, I see ulterior motives. In light of the information outlined so far in this book, it would appear that the FDA and USDA (United States Department of Agriculture) are constantly on both ends of a system that seems to both create and feed its own problems, leaving the average citizen stuck in the gears.

Economic Status: Contributing to Illness?

Before proceeding any farther, let's add yet another layer to our investigation. The USDA coins the phrase "food insecurity" to describe a household that has "difficulty in consistently obtaining adequate food because of limited economic resources for food." In July 2017, the USDA released a report connecting food insecurity with chronic disease among working-age adults. The study outlined the connection between limited economic means and ten chronic conditions identified as concerns by the CDC (Centers for Disease Control and Prevention). These conditions included hypertension, coronary heart disease (CHD), hepatitis, stroke, cancer, asthma, diabetes, arthritis, chronic obstructive pulmonary disease (COPD), and kidney disease, and were specifically targeted as an investigation within the average working age adult, because of the diseases "prevalence, cost, morbidity, and preventability."[51] The startling link present with all ten chronic conditions was food insecurity.

The report stated, "Extensive literature has examined the associations between food security and health, almost all of it showing the strong correlation between food insecurity and negative health outcomes."[52] Findings noted a significant difference in the rate of chronic illness in households where food security was very low. In fact, the highest percentage of probability for chronic illness was found within the households that showed lowest food security.

This means the USDA recognizes and is concerned with the fact that households who cannot afford to keep a consistent, adequate food supply are subject to chronic illness, more so than households who can afford to have the cabinets always stocked with a healthy, nutritious, adequate supply of food.

An even more recent report conducted by the USDA in August 2017 showed that those participating in SNAP (Supplemental Nutrition Assistance Program), after factoring in the amount of assistance received, still spent on average less money per person on food than other American households. Additionally, at-home food spending was a larger percentage of money spent on food. This means that households participating in food-assistance programs on average are eating at restaurants less often and, overall, are spending less money on food. The report states that the program "is designed to increase the food purchasing power of program participants. This, in turn, should increase their ability to achieve a nutritious diet and attain food security—having enough for an active, healthy life."[53] The report goes on to talk about the food spending pattern:

> We find that average daily food expenditures of SNAP households are substantially higher on the day of…benefit receipt than during the rest of the month. Expenditures then declined fairly rapidly over the two days after receipt and level off during the remainder of the…benefit month…. However, it is important to note that SNAP households may be able to smooth their food consumption over the month by making a large shopping trip right after their benefit receipt and slowly drawing down their food stores over the course of the month.[54]

What we gain from connecting all this information is the knowledge that those who are struggling financially and are food insecure are also then more prone to diseases and chronic illness. The lack of consistent nutrition is depriving their bodies of the ability to stay healthy. These people spend less money on food and less than other average Americans at restaurants. We can gather from the spike in grocery purchases on the day SNAP benefits are distributed the probability that, on top of being impoverished and/or food insecure, these families are also likely eating a lot of processed foods. Think about it this way: If you only received grocery money once a month (*not* a circumstance limited to those on SNAP assistance), you would be very unlikely to buy a lot of fresh produce or organic food. You would be looking for items with a longer shelf life, and you would want to get the most for your money. These goals point to cereals, crackers, boxed dinner kits, and other foods laden with preservatives. The only fresh items you might be inclined to buy would be what you could freeze or eat immediately. People at this point aren't likely as concerned with ingredients as they are with acquiring the food and making sure it is affordable and shelf-stable enough to last until the next SNAP disbursement. This is another level on which the low-income person is vulnerable to disease, and it's one more reason many people fear they cannot afford to eat organically.

Between 1999 and 2010, the USDA noted that food purchasing patterns were most effectively determined by changes in food pricing and total food expenditure, citing that "Americans are purchasing more processed foods because of those foods' declining market prices relative to their less processed counterparts."[55] The report then stated that the decline in the number of foods being prepared from scratch at home can also be attributed to the fact that more Americans are working and have less time to prepare food. While the report acknowledged that advertising played a big role in the spike in sales of fast-food meals and snacks, the astounding results showed that basic cooking ingredients comprised less than 25 percent of the average household's food budget. More frequently purchased were partially prepared meals and snacks, with the most convenient foods at the top of the occurrence list.

The case I'm making here is vast and extensive enough to become its own separate book. Suffice it to say that the busier and more economically challenged we are, the greater our propensity to purchase and eat the food that is making us sick. But for each passing day we don't realize we're sick, many of us count it as a small success and wake up the next morning to do it again. As stated before, many of us realize that there could be a ticking timebomb of health somewhere inside us, but for each day that passes without visible or currently diagnosed symptoms, we remain in our usual grind, hopeful we may dodge the proverbial bullet.

Your Body IS Reacting to Your Food

Our bodies give us signals we, sadly, often ignore. We tend to treat symptoms with quick fixes or medications when there is an underlying problem. Often it takes a physical ailment so painful or debilitating that we can't function to get us to stop and pay any attention at all. Even at that, often, we take a sick day to visit our doctor, obtain some sort of symptom-masking prescription drug, and jump straight back into our regular habits within a day or two. The only time we are pressed to dig deeper and look for the root of the problem is when the issue simply refuses to go away.

We fail to recognize that many of the issues our bodies manifest, though sometimes silenced (albeit temporarily) by medications, spring from dietary neglect. We live such busy lifestyles that often we don't pay attention to our bodies' signals. We ignore the mounting symptoms as they get louder and louder. By the time we stop to investigate, we have a much bigger problem on our hands than we would have had if only we had taken the time to address the source of the problem.

The results of dietary mistreatment of our bodies can be subtle at first. They can show up as symptoms we often blow off as simple aging: a fading complexion, brittle hair or hair loss, facial wrinkles, and oral health issues such as tooth decay or breakage, tooth loss, or swollen or bleeding gums. Although many of these signs are connected to aging, they have also been linked to deficiencies of elements such as protein, essential fatty acids, carotenoids, tocophernols, and flavonoids, or nutrients such as vitamins A, C, D, and E, as well as zinc and iron. Some of these issues have likewise been directly connected to poor diet habits, such as lack of fresh fruits and vegetables and unreasonably high sugar intake.

Another warning sign that our bodies are not receiving proper nutrition is easily dismissed as aging: problems with memory and concentration. Many people don't even know what omega-3 fatty acids are, let alone be able to tell you whether they are consuming an adequate amount to support brain function. Without it, our cognitive brain development suffers throughout all life stages. Likewise, these symptoms indicate that one's diet may contain far too many carbohydrates and lacking in protein. With my own illness, there were times that I would suffer from "brain fog," which I assumed was my age catching up to me. In addition, over time, the dying brain cells from an overabundance of excitotoxins can interrupt brain function as well.

Easy bruising, slow healing of cuts and bruises, or easy infection of wounds are also signs that your body is not receiving proper nutrition. Because so many of us are so busy and work so hard, it's easy to dismiss cuts and bruises as unimportant casualties of a busy lifestyle. Many of us have cuts or bruises that we can't account for and don't know how long we've had. Again, our bodies' condition becomes a casualty of a lifestyle that makes no time for proper care. When we see and experience these symptoms, we should know that we are suffering from a lack of calories, proteins, and micronutrients.

The immune system is also a big indicator of our overall health. Vitamins A, C, and E, as well as zinc, selenium, iron, and folic acid are key to maintaining healthy immune systems. Chronic infections of sinuses and ears, or other ailments such as cold and flu, often signal a bigger problem beneath the surface. If you are constantly on antibiotics, perhaps you should investigate the root reason.

Fatigue is another sign that our bodies are missing something important. The ironic thing about this symptom is that it can exacerbate the other ones. For example: I feel fatigued because my diet is poor. My other symptoms, such as low concentration and a weakened immune system, are worse because of my fatigue. As my body becomes more depleted, I feel even more fatigued, which further feeds these other issues. This becomes another cycle that simply cannot be treated without proper nutrition. Many people are happy to try to get more sleep, but they are missing the key ingredient that will enable their sleep to effectively help their bodies. Fatigue often suggests a diet overloaded with excessive carbohydrates and lacking in protein and vitamin C. It also indicates a taxed adrenal system, leading to a more serious health issue, such as the one I had.

The Cycle of Sickness

Because of the toxic ingredients in our food and the lack of nutrition provided by it, it is not abnormal for a person these days to be both obese and malnourished at the same time. This creates a dual polarization within the body: We simultaneously become prone to diseases associated with being overweight as well as suffer the health problems of the underfed. The result is a self-perpetuating cycle, and the farther in this wrong direction we travel, the harder it is to regain control over our health. In the next chapter, I will outline an overview of some of the common surface issues that spring from our food choices and how the cycle of illness affects our bodies in the long term.

6

You Could Already Be Sick

Check Yourself before You Wreck Yourself

One of the biggest contributing factors to our health problems today is the simple fact that we eat far too much food (as well as the wrong types) that contains toxic ingredients. Without even realizing it, most Americans are overeating at every meal. This means many of us are unknowingly destroying our health at a rapid pace.

Recent studies show that even short-term splurges such as those done on vacation or over holidays can trigger reactions within the body that cause overeating to become a habit. This is because the body's mechanisms that metabolize food go into overdrive when we overeat. In a rush to try to process the excess load that is pressed onto the body's metabolic and hormonal system, the body responds by rushing the food into stored fat. As the body is overloaded with food, the pancreas produces extra insulin to stabilize the bloodstream's sugar levels by removing excess sugar. Unfortunately, by the time the brain has caught up and sent the "all-clear" signal to the pancreas, allowing the system to return to normal, too much sugar has been removed, creating a low blood sugar incident of sorts, and contributing to the brain fog, sleepiness, dizziness, or even depression that follows. Have you ever experienced that "afternoon slump" that hits at about 2 or 3 PM? Many of us solve that problem by eating a quick, sugary "pick-me-up." Problem solved? Nope, problem repeated, because this resets the cycle. However, by the time the next slump hits in the early evening, we just tell ourselves, "Wow, I'm sleepy. It's been a long day."

This eating pattern also creates malfunction within the stomach, which begins to send mixed signals about whether it is actually full. This happens because the stomach has a neurological tissue at the top that signals the brain to stop eating when it is full. When we constantly overeat, this tissue begins to send erratic, inaccurate signals to the brain. At this point, you might be thinking, "But I never overeat, so I'm fine." Maybe, but the issue with this neurological pathway is that it stops sending the "full" signal. So, if you are overeating, you likely won't even know until you hit an extreme level of over-intake in one sitting. This is worse if you are drinking ice-cold drinks with your meal. The chilled effect the cold beverage has on this pathway causes your stomach to contract and send additional misinformation to the brain, making the brain even less likely to realize that you are indeed full. Because of the contracting of the stomach, it then sends the food into the gastrointestinal tract sooner than it is ready to, overloading the gut and making you feel hungry again sooner.

Chronic overindulgence creates strong urges to snack (not to mention the brain's addiction to excitotoxins), and the overload of foods (that are often sugary or processed) elevates the body's sugar levels, contributing to diabetes. Further, as we consume excess calories in response to these cravings and urges, truckloads of harmful chemicals in the form of junk food or even seemingly healthy snacks are still being ingested, contributing to gut issues and heart problems, or even feeding cancer within the body. The excess weight then contributes even more extensively to physical and emotional health problems, further propelling the downward spiral. As the body becomes addicted to carbs, it begins to rely on the constant influx to stay energetic and fight depression because of the fluctuation in sugars—a cycle that repeats. The excessive carbs then fuel the mind fog, memory problems, and depression, often leading us to look to more food to bring us back up, even though we don't realize we are both perpetuating and feeding this vicious, dangerous sequence. Whether we realize it or not, our bodies respond to what we are eating.

The way we Americans have learned to eat is unreliable at best. Let's again imagine that the body is a machine that has been entrusted to our care. What is our maintenance system? If you left your machine in another person's care and came back to find the maintenance, the addition of necessary fluids, and the care schedule as erratic as the way we typically treat our bodies, what would you say to that person? Let's be honest: I'd be angry. In general, we have failed our bodies. We have no set regimen of nutrients going in and no mandated schedule for when those nutrients are introduced. Many of us have no set eating schedule. We just eat whatever we want, whenever we want. This lack of schedule and structure causes our erratic dietary habits and contributes to chronic overeating.

Overeating Leads to Obesity...

It isn't necessary to explain that overeating leads to obesity, as that is obvious and well known. I will bring to your attention, however, that a recent study showed that the percentage of obese children and teenagers in the world grew tenfold between 1975 and 2016.[56] The double whammy is that many of these children also maintained signs of malnutrition, despite their hefty size. Researchers in *The Lancet* medical journal wrote: "If post-2000 trends continue, child and adolescent obesity is expected to surpass moderate and severe underweight by 2022."[57]

The study shows that the population now includes nearly 125 million obese boys and girls worldwide, while the underweight population numbers approximately 190 million. This means that while world hunger is still an epidemic, obesity is catching up fast. Since obesity comes with the increased risk of such diseases as diabetes, we stand to see health issues escalate unless we turn these statistics around. Most cases of diabetes can be prevented or reversed through diet. This means that if we can intervene on the issue of obesity, we can cut further disease off before it has a chance to take root in younger generations. Overweight children are also at heightened risk for complications beyond obesity, such as developmental problems or stunted growth, if they are additionally malnourished.

Which Leads to Diabetes...

Let's look at a comparison of sugar consumption from a recent article on the subject: In 1822, the average American consumed 45 grams of sugar every five days.[58] This is basically the amount of sugar in one soft drink being consumed over nearly a week. In 2012, the average American consumed 756 grams of sugar over the course of five days.[59] This is nearly seventeen times the amount of sugar we consumed in the year 1822, equaling approximately 130 pounds of sugar per individual each year! Further still, this shocking number only refers to *sugar*. It doesn't begin to touch on the amount of dangerous sugar substitutes we consume on a regular basis (eight hundred million pounds of aspartame is estimated to have been consumed by Americans since the 1980s[60]), further compromising our health. Sugar is absorbed into the body in two ways: It can either be (1) converted into energy or (2) stored as fat. In moderation (such as the amount consumed back in 1822), our bodies can keep up with the influx of sugar and convert it to energy without becoming overloaded and converting it to fat. This isn't the case with the excess amounts of sugar consumed by modern-day Americans. The problem is exacerbated by the fact that many of us live sedentary lifestyles, while simultaneously consuming these increasingly excessive amounts of sugar. Because of this, excess sugar is taken in is not burned as energy, and the body does not create enough demand for energy manufactured from its food intake. Our bodies literally cannot keep up with the constant incoming supply. As sugar is ingested, the pancreas releases insulin to attempt to deal with the incoming sugar now entering the bloodstream. When an overabundance of sugar is introduced at one time to the bloodstream (an occurrence during most American meals today), the pancreas responds by releasing too much insulin in an effort to deal with this excessive sugar and restore balance. But, as explained previously, by the time the pancreas receives the signal that it can stop producing insulin, it has already overproduced, resulting in a crash. When we experience this crash, then eat a sugary snack as a "boost," we create the erratic, roller-coaster style pattern of sugar polarity that eventually trains the body to malfunction where insulin and sugar are concerned, resulting in the development of diabetes.

And Cancer...

Recent studies show that cancers such as brain cancer, multiple myeloma, cancer of the esophagus, postmenopausal breast cancer, and cancers of the thyroid, gallbladder, stomach, liver, pancreas, kidney, ovaries, uterus, and colon are all linked to obesity.[61] One report stated that four in ten cases of cancers occurred in obese patients. Dr. Lisa Richardson of the CDC's Division of Cancer Prevention and Control stated that early evidence suggests that losing weight can decrease the risk for certain types of cancer. In the year 2014 alone, over 630,000 cases of cancer with obesity present were diagnosed in America. "Excluding colon cancer, the rate of obesity-related cancer increased by 7 percent between 2005 and 2014. During the same time, the rates of non-obesity-related cancers dropped, the findings showed."[62] Key findings further included that 55 percent of all cancers in women and 24 percent of all cancers in men were connected to obesity.

Those conducting the study clarified that obesity was not stated as the *cause* of the cancers and that the connection was still being explored; however, the World Cancer Research Fund estimated that excess body weight, excess alcohol, physical inactivity, and poor nutrition were responsible for at least 20 percent of all cancers in the United States.

"Healthy" People at Risk

At this point, you may be thinking that your own health has not been compromised. *After all,* you may be thinking, *I am not overweight, and I work out regularly. This problem doesn't apply to me.*

But it might.

The phrase "metabolically obese normal weight," or MONW, is described by the American Diabetes Association to apply to people who are:

> ...not obese on the basis of height and weight, but who, like people with overt obesity, are hyperinsulinemic, insulin-resistant, and predisposed to type 2 diabetes, hypertriglyceridemia, and premature coronary heart disease...[and that] such metabolically obese, normal-weight (MONW) individuals are very common in the general population and that they probably represent one end of the spectrum of people with the insulin resistance syndrome.[63]

In a nutshell, this condition renders the body of a thin person similar to that of an obese one, except that the person's signs of obesity are all beneath the skin. Amazingly, studies have shown that one in four adult individuals and four out of ten teenagers are carrying this ticking timebomb[64] and don't yet know it. This condition can lead to the same health problems as obesity, which makes it even more dangerous, because the victim is unsuspecting. *Further,* when diabetes kicks in, it is twice as likely to result in death for MONW individuals.

Dr. Mark Hyman said of MONW, "Insulin is the real culprit here— it is the fat storage hormone. It stores belly fat and leads to hormonal and metabolic changes that cause muscle loss and inflammation, furthering the vicious cycle of pre-diabetes or Type 2 diabetes— whether you are skinny or fat."[65]

MONW is just another byproduct of unhealthy diet. People who aren't necessarily gaining weight because of the toxins they are taking in might just have a more efficient metabolism that others who are obese. But lack of obesity does not guarantee health and long life.

In addition to the possibility that a person can be manifesting the risks associated with obesity or MONW, there is still the added risk factor that even our "whole foods" are contaminated.

How's Your Mind?

A story ran in October 2017 about a young couple about to deliver their first child when their world was suddenly devastated. The young father, who had been working long hours and commuting, suffered a brain hemorrhage and was forced to undergo life-saving brain surgery.[66] This event launched a series of medical complications such as seizures, strokes, and further brain surgeries. What was the culprit behind this terrible event? The excessive consumption of energy drinks. At this point, the reader may argue that it is a well-established fact that energy drinks are dangerous. And this is true. This story represents the extreme of what can happen when these toxic elements are introduced to our bodies in excess amounts.

However, there are lower levels at which our brains are affected by the chemicals we ingest every day. As I've already said, it's typical to ignore symptoms and continue with our current habits until something escalates that demands repair. We already established that many of the chemicals we ingest are perfectly capable of crossing the blood-brain barrier. It is important to understand how these elements affect our brain's chemistry and create results that can ripple into every part of our lives.

Allow me to return your attention to excitotoxins. The most common one is MSG, although it isn't the only source of these dangerous ingredients. Remembering that MSG dates back as early as 1908, we know this means that every adult in society today could be (and likely is) suffering from the effects of too many excitotoxins. Dr. Cathie Lippman, founder of the Lippman Center for Optimal Health, adds another layer to the alarm by revealing this scary truth about excitotoxins: "The younger the child, the greater the potential damage. This is particularly significant when we consider how many pregnant women get these chemicals in the processed foods they eat."[67]

We've already established the general danger of excitotoxins in their ability to cross the blood-brain barrier and affect the general chemistry of the brain. Remember, these ingredients, providing no benefit other than a heightened sense of pleasure via the taste buds, cause a series of erratic signals to be fired around the brain. Shortly after this experience, cells within the brain die that the body is unable to regenerate. Many of the ingredients that will be discussed in this book are proven to encourage hyperactivity or throw the blood sugar out of balance, creating the "highs" and "lows" of the pre-diabetic roller coaster. In general, the physical price that our bodies pay because of our food's flavor is steep indeed.

But how far out do the effects of these ingredients really go? In my research, I ran across a startling connection that we must not ignore. When Elizabeth Armstrong of the *Christian Science Monitor* wrote this report in 2004, it was a relatively new fact: "While antidepressants and other mood-altering drugs have long been prescribed to adolescents, the fastest-growing group using such medication is children under age 5."[68]

Between 1998 and 2002, the number of children taking antidepressants doubled. I wish I could say that this was an isolated story, or even that Elizabeth Armstrong was wrong. But sadly, it appears that this era marked the beginning of a new trend. Children ages 5 years and younger are now the fastest-growing demographic using antidepressants! Particularly alarming is that an increasing number of prescriptions are being written by medical doctors, not psychiatrists. Instead of turning to investigation about a child's behavior—such as evaluating home lives, activity levels, school setting, diet, or even deferring to counseling—many medical doctors are diagnosing first and asking questions later. Sadly, some doctors are even encouraged to prescribe medication since the parents cannot afford counseling.[69] Other parents opt to medicate because they are unable to be home full-time to enforce a structured regimen that could potentially correct the child's behavior. Parents of children who are lashing out often readily agree to these medications for a few reasons:

1. Assuming bad behavior means the child is unhappy, parents want to relieve the behavior so that they will believe their child is happy.

2. When a child is behaving badly, it usually results in punishment, either at home or at school. Rather than let a child live in "disapproval" that might affect his or her self-esteem, parents allow the child to take medications to prevent the behavior that gets them into trouble in the first place.

3. The parents are unaware of other routes they could take to address their child's behavior.

In 2010, The *X Factor* author K. J. Antonia reported:

Dr. Jane Luby, the professor and researcher whose work in support of creating such a diagnosis… [diagnosis such as "adjustment disorder with depressed mood" or "depressive disorder not otherwise specified" in children as young as 18 months] suggests that as many as 84,000 preschoolers could be clinically depressed. That's a decent number of new customers for the pharmaceutical companies.[70]

In her article, she mentioned a child who, though just 18 months, had been on such severe medication as "the antipsychotic Risperdal, the antidepressant Prozac, to sleeping medicines, and one for attention-deficit disorder.[71]"

Don't misunderstand my point: Awareness regarding depression and intervention for suicide prevention are very important. But are our children *really* depressed in these kinds of numbers, at these young ages? Or is something else involved? Perhaps an ingredient in our food is causing their brains to fire erratically with stimulation and then "crash." Adults experiencing these sensations have a better understanding of what is happening to their bodies, even if the only names they have for it are "sugar high" and "carb crash." Adults are used to being tired because they work a lot. When they're grumpy, they attribute their mood to a bad day. When they're happy or energetic, they attribute their high spirits to having enjoyed a good night's sleep. Our children have no such communication skills, especially as young as 18 months! But from the time they cut their first tooth, most of their systems are being bombarded with ingredients that neither their bodies nor their brains are equipped to process. Perhaps the brain of the child has been overloaded with excitatory neurotransmitter substances, to a level five to twenty times higher than the typical chemistry make-up the body would maintain.[72]

Judi Clements, chief executive of the Mental Health Foundation, stated:

While early treatment for depression is important at any age, the foundation doesn't want to see children being given powerful psychiatric drugs. Antidepressants have potentially severe side-effects and we fear the safety and efficacy of giving them to children; there has been little research on the effects of such medication on the very young. What we would emphasize for a child's mental wellbeing and development is the importance of a supportive environment and sound parenting.

The long-term side effects of psychotropic and psychiatric drugs have been shown to manifest in such symptoms as psychosis, hallucinations, mania, depression, mood swings, and depersonalization, and can even double the risk of suicide. These drugs can also contribute to the occurrence of heart attacks and strokes, and can increase the probability of chronic illness. Because the side effects usually show up within the realms of mood swings, depression, psychosis, or hallucinations, they're often misconstrued as more symptoms of the root problem. This leads people to believe the medication prescribed isn't addressing the source, or that the original mental condition is elevating. This causes, in many cases, a diagnosis of mental illness and prescriptions are increased or intensified. This cycle begins to perpetuate itself as the new, more intense medication or increased dosage of the current medication is administered over time.

As I stated before, I'm glad awareness for mental illness has evolved over past decades. But it is important to understand the difference in *true mental illness* and *food-induced symptoms*. Studies show that over their lifetimes, almost 50 percent of Americans will develop what could technically be diagnosed as a mental illness.[73] Part of the reason is that "awareness" has evolved, *some of which* is wonderful. But, on the other hand, symptoms created by our response to toxic food can cause behaviors that may not have been considered a mental illness in previous years, but qualify as being indicative of a mental illness now. It seems that there is a disorder for nearly every type of human emotion now, whereas generations ago, only the emotional extremes were addressed. The good-versus-evil nature of this "awareness" is a vast topic, so for our purposes, I will merely remind the reader what Gwen Olsen had to say about campaigns that raise "awareness" advocated by the pharmaceutical world:

> Pharmaceutical companies are not charities. They are looking for a return on their investment. Overall, these programs are just well-disguised marketing campaigns designed to increase consumer awareness, thereby increasing drug sales for that disease. The success of the latest marketing ploy of promoting diseases in lieu of drugs is self-evident.[74]

Children in public school are being profiled under the heading of "social and emotional learning."[75] While there are many good things about this type of monitoring, and many of the people practicing it have good intentions, know without a doubt that your children's moods, behaviors, social struggles, and learning difficulties are being profiled under assessments such as the Devereux Student Strengths Assessment. Questions on the test are meant to identify the child's strengths and weaknesses in both academic and social settings.

About this type of profiling, Dr. Aida Cerundolo of the *Wall Street Journal* said, "The mental-health information [that] teachers are now obtaining, storing, and tracking.... Is equally as sensitive as that which is collected in a pediatrician's office."[76]

Piecing this together, we have an upcoming generation of children who have, since *before birth,* been fed stimulants that are known to enter brain chemistry and alter brain function. These ingredients are without doubt connected to many behavioral disorders, contributing to the premature prescribing of behavioral medications at an insanely young age. Many of these children now on medication (the largest upcoming demographic taking antidepressants and other psychiatric drugs) are now being profiled by a system that has adjusted its "awareness" to qualify 50 percent of the population as being mentally ill.

The long-term implication of this cycle alarms me. If 50 percent of our society could be diagnosed with mental illness, what will happen if the laws change regarding the *rights of the mentally ill*? Will we still be allowed to purchase guns? Will we still be able to vote? What about our right to a fair and speedy trial? Is there a potential for us to be placed in care homes or elsewhere against our will? I realize this may seem like a stretch, but recall George Orwell's futuristic novel *1984*. "Big brother is watching you"[77] became the catchphrase to remind characters in the story that they were under constant surveillance. I'm certain it made for a good read at the time, but many people then would have denied there would ever be any merit to it.

It is possible that the healthcare system is overwhelmed and needs repair. It is also possible that, as a society, we are being attacked, suffering an onslaught from all directions. Those who are too busy feel they don't have time to change their situation. Those who cannot afford to "buy organic" feel powerless as well. Some are too fatigued, sick, or even depressed to take the initiative. But, we can no longer afford to be silenced as a society, too sick or too mentally unstable to act on our own behalf. For up-and-coming generations, it is up to us to make a change in the way we handle our food.

We're seeing a new trend of consumer vigilance on the rise. It is possible to take back our power. Our problem is not that we are powerless, our *problem is that we believe ourselves to be so*. Again, that very first ingredient is the most dangerous, toxic, of them all. If you have any lingering doubt that this is everyone's problem, it will likely be eliminated within the next chapter.

7

This Is Everyone's Problem

Control oil and you control nations;
control food and you control the people.
—Henry Kissinger

There is nobody who won't eventually be affected by what is happening with our food crisis. There is a timebomb in 80 percent of American guts, ticking down to an inevitable health catastrophe if the warning that we must change our lifestyle goes unheeded. Those who think they're not affected simply haven't seen the impact on their own personal lives—just yet. Additionally, *our food supply* has been infiltrated by powers that cannot be trusted to place the human race's well-being at top priority, and there is no "back-up plan" for when the food being produced is finally so corrupt that we can no longer turn a blind eye. This problem is *everyone's* problem, because it will eventually catch up with *all of us.*

Lack of Regulations = Contamination of Food Supply

When we trace our food back to its origin, it becomes apparent that many conglomerates are owned by a handful of large corporations. Much of the food sold throughout our country comes from surprisingly few sources. What began as small, local businesses buying and selling locally generated food have become commercial, globalized commerce. Food manufacturers that buy in extremely large quantities operate in such high volumes that they control how their own products are manufactured, marketed, and sold. In addition, because of their buying power, they have a tremendous influence on how the market standard is set on such products across the board. This means that when we shop, we are probably buying products that have been built according to these corporate buyers' specs. For example, since McDonald's is the highest-volume purchaser of both ground beef and potatoes in America,[78] its volume and needs dictate a large part of how ground beef and potato productions are operated. The problem is that the large corporations our food is being manufactured *for* do not have the same needs as consumers. We're looking for a healthy, reliable, and safe product. They're looking for inexpensive, mass-produced goods they can sell at a high profit yield and prepare with quick and easy methods. This very business model feeds the notion that health, quality, and safety do not come first and result in manufacturing shortcuts such as added chemicals, contamination and sanitation issues, and the strangling out of the small farmer.

On top of all of this, we've already established that the FDA can't keep up with all the necessary legislation and inspection that it would require to ensure that all our food sources are safe. The longer we allow this trend to continue, the more lackadaisical the governing of our food quality will become, leaving our entire food supply increasingly and perpetually vulnerable unless we make significant changes, demanding that better protection for the consumer begins now. This will only be done through public outcry, consumer vigilance, and boycott of destructive foods. Even if the current situation isn't necessarily *bothering you yet* (though it should be), understand that, considering the direction we are heading, it's only a matter of time before the lack of consumer protection affects each of us.

Conglomerate Farmers vs. Small Farmers

To explain the plight of the small farmer, we must start at the beginning. Donald L. Barlett and James B. Steele of Vanity Fair Online sum up this story's setting in the following excerpt:

> For centuries—millennia—farmers have saved seeds from season to season: they planted in the spring, harvested in the fall, then reclaimed and cleaned the seeds over the winter for re-planting the next spring. Monsanto has turned this ancient practice on its head.
>
> Monsanto developed G.M. seeds that would resist its own herbicide, Roundup, offering farmers a convenient way to spray fields with weed killer without affecting crops. Monsanto then patented the seeds. For nearly all of its history the United States Patent and Trademark Office had refused to grant patents on seeds, viewing them as life-forms with too many variables to be patented. "It's not like describing a widget," says Joseph Mendelson III, the legal director of the Center for Food Safety, which has tracked Monsanto's activities in rural America for years.
>
> Indeed not. But in 1980 the U.S. Supreme Court, in a five-to-four decision, turned seeds into widgets, laying the groundwork for a handful of corporations to begin taking control of the world's food supply. In its decision, the court extended patent law to cover "a live human-made microorganism." In this case, the organism wasn't even a seed. Rather, it was a Pseudomonas-

bacterium developed by a General Electric scientist to clean up oil spills. But the precedent was set, and Monsanto took advantage of it. Since the 1980s, Monsanto has become the world leader in genetic modification of seeds and has won 674 biotechnology patents, more than any other company, according to U.S. Department of Agriculture data.

Farmers who buy Monsanto's patented Roundup Ready seeds are required to sign an agreement promising not to save the seed produced after each harvest for re-planting, or to sell the seed to other farmers. This means that farmers must buy new seed every year. Those increased sales, coupled with ballooning sales of its Roundup weed killer, have been a bonanza for Monsanto.[79]

The aftermath of this "agricultural breakthrough" has been that farmers signed away their age-old, God-given right to save seeds from year to year. Seeds cannot be sold or shared, unused seeds must be disposed of at the end of each year, and new seeds must be purchased the following year to prevent violation of the agreement. Because centuries of good agriculture were founded on these very principles, counterintuitive and counterproductive practices have been required of farmers who previously never would have agreed to such practices.

Neighboring farms to these growers of Monsanto seed are compromised by transference of seed, which places the Monsanto seed grower and these neighboring innocent bystanders in the vulnerable position of being investigated by Monsanto for unauthorized sharing/selling/planting of seed. Transferring seed between neighboring farms is easy. Shared equipment, wind, and birds are only a few ways that seeds can be unintentionally relocated to nearby farms. If the seed is transmitted between farms, the farmer in violation can be sued by Monsanto, resulting in total loss of his farm's assets. This isolation of seed likewise isolates the farmers, creating a detriment to previously thriving farmer coop practices and tearing down the spirit of community that traditionally has been the small farmer's means of industry survival.

Farmers claim that a team of investigators sent out by Monsanto enforce their policies by scrutinizing seeds grown by anyone they suspect may be using their product in an unauthorized manner. Some farmers are intimidated by them, and some have reported their behavior as being shady or aggressive. Monsanto, once mainly a chemical company, has shifted its attention to the agricultural realm in recent years, and has grown to be one of the strongest powers behind our agricultural food supply. This means that when their investigative team finds a violation—founded or unfounded—by any small farmer, the farmer's financial resources usually dry up long before Monsanto's. Many would argue that Monsanto is not intimidating small farmers, while pointing out that cases rarely go to court. But this is because most small farmers, even when they try to fight for their rights, are bankrupt before their case even gets that far.

Monsanto's purchase of Calgene in the 1980s was only the beginning of its acquisitions, as Barlett and Steele went on to report:

> Even as the company is pushing its G.M. agenda, Monsanto is buying up conventional-seed companies. In 2005, Monsanto paid $1.4 billion for Seminis, which controlled 40 percent of the U.S. market for lettuce, tomatoes, and other vegetable and fruit seeds. Two weeks later it announced the acquisition of the country's third-largest cottonseed company, Emergent Genetics, for $300 million. It's estimated that Monsanto seeds now account for 90 percent of the U.S. production of soybeans, which are used in food products beyond counting. Monsanto's acquisitions have fueled explosive growth, transforming the St. Louis-based corporation into the largest seed company in the world.[80]

What Monsanto can't buy out, it closes through intimidation tactics. In the 1980s, GMO farming was completely new to American soil. By 2007, the total acres planted exceeded 142 million acres.[81] Ironically, the original draw of the small farmer to this seed was its ability to withstand the chemical Roundup. What would have previously destroyed crops is now being sprayed on the new, genetically modified crop that is able to withstand such a chemical. It goes without saying that neither the crop nor the chemical *should* be ingested by humans.

Many farmers initially lured in by this convenient way of farming have since come to regret their decision. Many feel as though they are under surveillance, as are their neighbors, to ensure that seeds aren't being transferred (purposely *or* unintentionally), and they believe that Monsanto won't hesitate to file lawsuits against them, accusing them of "knowingly, intentionally, and willfully" planting seeds in violation of Monsanto's patent rights.[82] Many farmers are approached by Monsanto's assertive investigators, who tell them that they are the subject of investigation even when the farmers deem the accusations are unfounded. Some farmers have reported acts of intimidation, such as threats to bring neighboring farms into the case or showing surveillance photos of the farmers to reveal that they have been followed by investigators. It is reported that they then insist that the farmer sign accompanying paperwork.[83]

A brief historical overview of Monsanto will remind the reader that this company, for a century, has introduced the world to one harmful chemical after another, many of which cause cancer, heart disease, liver damage, and damage to the reproductive, endocrine, and immune systems, and the chemicals also have terrible environmental consequences. Court documents going back to the 1950s show that Monsanto was likely aware of the harm caused by their products, but the company dodged these facts. We must remember exactly who we are dealing with: Monsanto's new stance of creating better agriculture to benefit the world, adopted in 2002, is a euphemism for saying they have found a new way to monopolize a lucrative industry at the cost of the people and environment.

Monsanto is also the developer of rBHG, a growth hormone used in dairy cows to increase milk delivery. When dairies opting not to treat their cows with this injected hormone began to advertise this fact with slogans such as "rBHG Free!" Monsanto attempted to petition legislation against such advertising, stating that is adversely reflected on dairies that *did* use the hormone. The ironic thing about this hormone's use is that while it is being marketed, the government continues to subsidize manufacturing of food materials made from surplus milk. This means that we do not *need* a production hormone in our dairy cows. We have an *excess* of it already. Additionally, cows treated with this hormone show signs of mastitis, lameness, uterus and birthing complications, digestive problems, and elevated body temperature. So *why* this push to introduce this chemical to our dairy cows? Why does Monsanto want this chemical in our food animals? And why is it so important to Monsanto that dairies not using it keep that information off their labels?

Another way the small farmer is under attack is through corporate buying. Stories like that of Karen and Mitchell Crutchfield are common enough, and go much like this:[84] A farmer growing poultry or cattle must constantly go up against corporations that can raise food animals in higher volumes, thus selling at prices so low that a smaller farm can't compete. Farmers who don't have a wide enough client base of customers willing to pay higher prices for locally raised products are often tempted by the "security" offered by high-profile, corporate buyers. However, once they enter contracts with these companies, they are subject to mandated "upgrades" demanded by these high-paying clients. Many farmers borrow against their farms or homes to fund these demanded upgrades (things like computer systems, equipment, or animal housing facilities) only to have requirements change soon thereafter, necessitating new purchases and additional loans. When new demands are made, often farmers are replacing or upgrading perfectly operational equipment until they can no longer afford to take on additional debt to fund these corporate demands. Attempted negotiations by farmers, such as proposing that they upgrade half the farm one year and the other half the next, meet with threats to withdraw purchase agreements.[85] Demands must be met in their entirety to keep contract with the corporate buyers. The farmer's refusal to comply likewise results in threats of cancellation of his or her contract. Unable to afford this loss of business, farmers are left with two options: 1) take on further debt to make demanded upgrades or purchases, or 2) risk losing the farm by sacrificing the business they have invested so much in and now rely on due to the debt they have taken on. Farmers who try to fight for their rights often lose their farms. Dan Fesperman and Kate Shatzkin of the *Baltimore Sun* summed up this dilemma when they wrote about chicken farmers who lost their battle against ConAgra: "Farmers sold their chicken houses at salvage prices. Four eventually signed with other poultry firms in the region, but only after their chicken houses sat empty for two years, incurring huge losses. Several of the rest are saddled with debts they'll be paying for decades for chicken houses they'll never again use."[86]

If You Can't Beat 'Em, Join 'Em?

For many farmers, the competition from corporate farms is too much to keep up with. The other option, joining forces with the corporations, is a trap that can, and often does, bankrupt these individuals and their families. This scenario leaves our last few independent farmers still out there, hanging on in a vulnerable position. They are likely selling at higher prices than their corporate counterparts, and probably don't have the distribution outlets of their competitors. The small farms operate with integrity and meet needs in specific niches of the industry. These farmers need our support so they can remain strong in an industry where they are outnumbered and undersold. Your dollars, in boycott, may not be enough to hurt a conglomerate food industry, but, spent in the right places, that money is enough to begin a change for good. Support your local farmer every chance you get!

What's in Our Meat?

For decades (despite that the European Union stopped buying US meat in 1985 due to hormone use[87]), hormones have been used in meat production to increase yield at a faster rate. Although many argue that these chemicals are safe, a closer look causes us to be wary. Many of these substances are similar or identical to elements contained in our own pharmaceutical drugs, and many have also demonstrated frightening side effects on animals when tested.

Defenders of the use of hormones and antibiotics maintain that the levels contained in ingested meat are low enough that they are not toxic to humans. They also argue that the level of these elements contained in meat is much lower because many of these chemicals are administered by a subcutaneous implant, usually in the ear, rather than being ingested by the animal. The implant then releases the chemicals into the animal's body over time. Advocates of these chemicals say that oral ingestion results in a smaller absorption rate. Further arguments in favor of hormone use state that many of these chemicals are "structurally identical to that produced endogenously in human beings,"[88] meaning that because our bodies make these chemicals or "structurally identical" matches for these chemicals, it must be safe to ingest more. This is like the argument we've already made for glutamate. The body makes what it needs as it needs it, but that doesn't make it safe to ingest foreign sources of it in large quantities.

While it isn't possible to give a complete list of all antibiotics and hormones used in food animals, a few are listed below to make you aware of the types of chemicals that we can encounter in products from food animals.

rBGH (Recombinant Bovine Growth Hormone)—This synthetic hormone, used by dairy farmers to boost their production of milk, has been used for more than two and a half decades in the US, but it is not allowed in the European Union, Canada, and certain other countries.[89] One of the biggest debates surrounding this substance is that its use has been linked to higher rates of mastitis within the cows it is administered to, leading to higher residuals of antibiotics in the final product.[90] In addition, milk from cows that have been treated with this synthetic hormone "has higher levels of insulinlike growth factor-1. IFG-1 is a hormone that helps cells grow, but it can also increase the risk of cancerous cells forming, according to the American Cancer Society. High levels of IFG-1 in the human body might raise the risk of certain types of cancers, such as breast, prostate, and colon."[91] Despite the assurances of many farms still using rBGH, many people avoid purchasing products associated with it, causing large corporations such as Walmart to respond by presenting rBGH-free alternatives for consumers to purchase.[92]

Estradiol—This is used alone or blended with testosterone to obtain weight gain and feed efficiency. This substance binds with intracellular receptors, particularly with females, to generate growth and encourage sexual maturity. A toxicological research report released by Hoseo University in 2010 said this:Estradiol has genotoxic potential by inducing micronuclei, aneuploidy, and cell transformation *in vitro*, and oxidative damage to DNA and DNA single-strand breakage *in vivo*.... In long-term studies of carcinogen 80 in mice and in rats, increased incidences of tumors were found in mammary and pituitary gland; the uterus, cervix, vagina, and testicles; and lymphoid organs and bone.... Malignant kidney tumors occurred in intact and castrated male hamsters and in ovariectomized female hamsters...estradiol 17 is a Group I carcinogen that has sufficient evidences for carcinogenicity to humans.... A result of its interaction with hormonal receptors because tumors largely occur in tissues possessing high levels of hormone receptors. Overall, estradiol is evaluated as a genotoxic carcinogen, however, it is necessary to consider that estradiol is a natural hormone synthesized in the human body and used as a human medicine.[93]

Progesterone—This chemical, like estradiol, is administered in the ear to promote weight gain and feed efficiency and to regulate the reproductive system. Also like estradiol, progesterone is believed to be less absorbent when ingested orally than when administered subcutaneously. In humans, this substance is used for hormone replacement therapy and sometimes contraception. Negative effects manifested when this was administered to female mice. Here is what the University of Hosco's Toxicological Research Report said about the results of this experiment:

> Progesterone was administered subcutaneously alone for five days beginning 36 h after birth causing ovary-dependent, persistent imaginal quantification and hyperplasia in the vaginal and cervical epithelia, and significantly higher incidence of mammary tumors in mammary tumor—virus bearing mice.... Increased incidences of ovarian, uterine, and mammary tumors in mice as well as mammary gland tumors in dogs.... These effects were regarded as hormone activity related.[94]

Other synthetic hormones used include Xenobiotic growth promoters such as Zeranol, Melengestrol, and Trenbolone Acetate. In studies involving mice, subjects manifested tumors in the anterior lobe of the pituitary gland due to estrogenic properties of Zeranol. Melengestrol showed a low acute level of toxicity after administered orally, although it is not considered an actual genotoxic chemical. It is linked to tumors in mice due to the increased release of Prolactin, and "induced reproductive toxicity as impaired pregnancy and parturition and greater pup loss in

Beagle dogs, and…exerted embryotoxic, feel toxic, and teratogenic effects including resorption, dead fetuses, visceral malformation, and incomplete skeletal ossification in rabbits."[95]

Trenbolone acetate, given in conjunction with estradiol or Zeranol:

> …induced liver hyperplasia in mice…. And islet-cell tumors of the pancreas in rats…. As a consequence of the hormonal activity…. In pigs… Induced hormonal effects involving decreased testosterone levels in the serum of male pigs; reductions in weight of the testes, ovaries, and uteri; atrophy of testicular interstitial cells; suppression of cyclic ovarian activity; absence of glandular development of the uterine endometrium; and lack of alveolar development and secretion in the mammary glands.[96]

While the argument in favor of using these drugs continues to be that oral ingestion causes an absorption rate so minuscule that there can be "no adverse effects" (an argument supported by the fact that desired results in animals are attained by administering these drugs subcutaneously into the ear of the animal), we can't help but wonder: If it were true that it was not orally absorbent, why would many of these chemicals be prescriptions for men and women dealing with hormonal issues, available in a pill, requiring a prescription from a doctor, and to be taken *orally*?

A recent study showed that antimicrobial drugs used in animals intended for food for human consumption led to increased drug resistance in humans.[97] The bottom line is that when unnecessary antibiotics are fed to animal crops for the mere purpose of higher yield and fewer casualties, the meat we eat passes those antibiotic qualities on to our systems as well. This has resulted in the increase of new and mutated strains of antibiotic-resistant infections in both livestock and people.

Of all antibiotics sold in the US, 80 percent are used on livestock. "According to the Environmental Working Group, 87 percent of tested meat samples (turkey, pork, beef, and chicken) were contaminated by at least one species of antibiotic-resistant bacteria."[98]

Since hormone use is prohibited in poultry, it might seem difficult to understand why a chicken breast purchased in 2017 is twice the size of a chicken breast purchased in 1950. A revealing article released in June 2017 by the Organic Consumers Association may shed some light:

> Three nonprofit groups filed suit today against Laurel, Miss.-based Sanderson Farms, Inc.… For falsely advertising products that contain a wide range of unnatural and in some cases prohibited substances, as "100% Natural." Substances include antibiotics, steroids, hormones and even a drug with hallucinogenic effects. The groups suing Sanderson are Organic Consumers Association (OCA), Friends of the Earth (FoE), and Center for Food Safety (CFS).[99]

This article highlights that food safety inspections conducted by the USDA "found 49 instances in which samples of Sanderson products tested positive for residues of synthetic drugs that are not '100% Natural.' Thirty-three percent of the 69 FSIS [Food Safety and Inspections Service] inspections, conducted in five states, uncovered residues that no reasonable consumer would consider 'natural.'"[100]

Within the results of this series of inspections, Sanderson was found in violation by means of antibiotics including chloramphenicol, a drug illegal for use with food animals. Ketamine was identified (a drug having hallucinogenic qualities), which is approved for use in beef and pork, not poultry. Also found were Ketoprofen (anti-inflammatory), Prednisone (steroid), Melengestrol Acetate and a beta agonist Ractopamine (both growth hormones prohibited in poultry), amoxicillin and penicillin (both antibiotics), and traces of abamectin and Emamectin (pesticides).

This story is alarming and comforting to me at the same time. I find it extremely disturbing that chicken was being sold as "100% Natural" (a label phrase not to be largely trusted, which we will discuss later in the book) while it was subjected to so many chemicals, many of which are illegal for use in poultry. At the same time, I am comforted that the USDA's Food and Safety Inspection Service (FSIS) inspections were able to detect these chemicals and alert proper authorities. I also find it encouraging that organic associations such as those involved in this case are willing to take action. Being on the lookout for cases like this can help us identify brands that are trustworthy—or not—and it also helps direct us to associations that we can follow for good leads regarding unwholesome organic food. It still falls on us shoppers to be our own vigilant guardians, but it's nice to know we're not alone.

In October 2017, Homeland Security News Wire released a story headlined: "Massive increase in antimicrobial use in animals to lead to widespread drug resistance in humans."[101] The article posed the issue that, unless policies were put into place to limit use of antibiotics within food animals, by 2030, 52 percent of our food animals will have been treated with antimicrobials. A frightening statement in the article was made by Emma Glennon, a Gates Scholar and PhD student at Cambridge's Department of Veterinary Medicine:

> Worldwide, animals receive almost triple the amount of antibiotics that people do, although much of this use is not medically necessary, and many new strains of antibiotic-resistant infections are now common in people after originating in our livestock. As global demand for meat grows and agriculture continues to transition from extensive farming and smallholdings to more intensive practices, the use of antimicrobials in food production will increasingly threaten the efficacy of these life-saving drugs.[102]

Recommendations resulting from this study involved creating a fee system requiring facilities to pay additional charges for antibiotics used on food animals. The hope behind this suggestion is that monies would be redirected into sanitation facilities and preventative measures, rendering antibiotics unnecessary.

The issue goes even deeper than this; only 20 percent of the antibiotics used in commercial farming are given to treating disease. The other 80 percent are administered for one of two reasons: (1) growth promotion or (2) disease prevention due to illnesses caused by unsanitary or overcrowded conditions. So, these chemicals are either used for commercial gain (which will catch up to us, since twenty-three thousand people die from antibiotic-resistant bugs, or "superbugs" each year[103]), or we are allowing these *living beings* to dwell in deplorable conditions that we don't correct and instead medicate. Many animals await their slaughter on a concrete slab, sitting in their own feces. Such an overuse of antibiotics in our food animals is an indicator that we have an underlying problem of either sanitation or greed, either of which should be addressed through something other than medication.

Beyond this, I feel it is wrong to turn a blind eye to this neglectful treatment of a living being. Think about it this way: If you *owned* that food animal and knew all along that its *entire life and death* would be spent in preparation for supplying you and your family with food, how would you treat that animal during its life? It's easy to forget the cost and eat food placed before us without considering that, more often than not, an animal had to die to give us that meal. It is my conviction that the animals that provide food for our families should be treated with respect and good husbandry during their lives here on earth.

Eat Your Veggies...

In addition to our meats being loaded with pharmaceuticals, we have the erosion within the nutritional density of our produce. Over the last fifty to seventy years, the mineral, vitamin, and protein content of our fruits and vegetables has dropped considerably. On top of the dangerous collection of eating habits that we as Americans have picked up, with the nutritional level of our food declining at a scary pace, we have traded nutrient-rich crops for higher-yield crops. We're raising fruits, vegetables, and grains in higher volumes, but they are depleted in vital nutrients such as vitamins, minerals, calcium, and protein content that our bodies need. Remember when you were young and your mom told you that you *had* to eat that broccoli because it was good for you? Today, that reasoning would hold less water than it did back when you were a child. In fact, I'm not sure *what* Popeye's status would be if he ate the spinach pulled from a modern can: This may be a sequel we do not want to see. And this very paradox of higher *quantities* of crops that are lower in nutrients perpetuates the cycle that while we have *more food available for consumption*, we are eating *food of lower overall quantity*. This fosters issues such as obese malnutrition, because what we really need is *less food consumed that is of better quality*.

At a glance, several reasons for this change within our crops readily surface: We've chosen to plant varieties based on their faster maturation and higher yields, and soil depletion is a huge culprit as well. "Modern intensive agricultural methods have strict increasing amounts of nutrients from the soil in which the food we eat grows," a *Scientific American* article reports. "Sadly, each successive generation of fast-growing, pest-resistant carrot is truly less good for you than the one before."[104]

Donald Davis, part of a team of researchers from the University of Texas at Austin's Department of Chemistry and Biochemistry, published a report in 2004 in the *Journal of the American College of Nutrition*, which stated that between the years of 1950 and 1999, forty-three fruit and vegetable varieties had seen "reliable declines" in protein, calcium, iron, phosphorus, vitamin C and vitamin B2.[105] Other elements noted as having declined were phytonutrients, antioxidants and vitamin A.

In addition to this study, Kushi Institute studies found that from 1975 to 1997, in twelve fresh vegetables, the following declines had taken place: 27 percent less calcium, 37 percent less iron, 21 percent less vitamin A, and 30 percent less vitamin C. Aadditionally, a study published in the *British Food Journal* showed the following declines in twenty vegetables: 19 percent less calcium, 22 percent less iron, and 14 percent less potassium.[106]

A hard copy of this report is alarming. Forty-three garden crop fruits and vegetables analyzed from USDA data reported in 1950, compared with a modern example of the same veggies, showed a disturbing decline in nearly all nutritional properties. The report noted that close modern equivalents were used, taking in to consideration size and other attributes of the mature product. Nutrient reductions in most of these garden crops were comparable to those previously mentioned, but the conclusion of the report states that the majority of dietary issues suffered by Americans is not a direct result of the nutritional decline in vegetables and fruits, but rather in the common overindulgence of fats, sugars, and grains, rendering even the degenerated garden crop a healthier option. After all, a slightly less nutritious vegetable is still better than a fatty, sugary diet. What disturbs me about this is the fact that these declines could continue if our farming and buying methods don't change, eventually rendering our produce nutritionally bankrupt. We must act while we have time. As it stands now, even individuals who are striving to do the best they can for their diets are affected by the changes taking place within the realms of our food production. When our fruits and veggies are declining in nutrients, the problem affects us all.

Furthermore, Marco Torres of *Signs of the Times Online* adds, "The important thing to note in these deficiencies is that these are exactly the deficiencies in a human being that lead to susceptibility to sickness, disorders and cancer. People who have osteoporosis are low in calcium and magnesium, people who have cancer are low in manganese. The list goes on and on."[107]

Another study also showed that edible, wild plants are often denser in nutrients than the ones we buy at the supermarket, which I find to have interesting implications. According to *New York Times* author Jo Robinson:

> Wild dandelions, one of the springtime treat for Native Americans, have seven times more phytonutrients than spinach, which we consider a "superfood." A purple potato native to Peru has 28 times more cancer–fighting anthocyanins then common russet potatoes. One species of Apple have a staggering 100 times more phytonutrients than the Golden Delicious displayed in our supermarkets.
>
> Were the people who foraged for these wild foods healthier than we are today? They did not live nearly as long as we do, but growing evidence suggests that they were much less likely to die from degenerative diseases, even the minority who lived 70 years and more. The primary cause of death for most adults, according to anthropologists, with injury and infections.[108]

The article goes on to explain that plants containing high levels of phytonutrients often have a bitter taste. The author makes the case that farmers over the years preferentially planted crops that had a sweeter, more palatable taste, thus ruling out some of the healthiest food sources that nature has had to offer. As soil depletion became an increasing concern and new breeds of crops were introduced for better flavor, the nutritional value of these crops declined. Could it be that the ones mankind left alone retained their nutritional value while we have been and continue to breed the nutrition completely out of certain ones that we "chose" at some point? I believe that is exactly what Robinson is alluding to.

Soil depletion is a reversible condition that can be improved upon if consumers will demand a different type of agricultural product. While it will not solve all the problems addressed in this book, it can certainly be a point of revolution. By insisting on higher-quality crops, we can begin to change the standard for food products across the board.

Damage to the Earth Affects Us All

The excessive use of pesticides contaminates soil and water sources, causing loss of biodiversity, destroying the natural enemies of pests, and reducing the nutritional value of food. The impact of such overuse also imposes staggering costs on national economies around the world.[109]

With our current food production trends in place, the toll our environment is taking will stay around for decades to come, even if we begin immediate change. Many agricultural companies claim that chemical-based agriculture is the only way to ensure that we can grow enough food to feed everybody. Others argue that we have enough food to feed the entire planet; but that the issue lies in inequality and distribution.[110] Regardless of what side of this argument we fall on, one thing is clear: Agricultural chemicals are dangerous for the environment. What's worse, they have been linked to "cancer, Alzheimer's and Parkinson's diseases, and disruption, developmental disorders and sterility.... Populations most at risk are farmers and agricultural workers."[111]

Perhaps the introduction of such chemicals into the agricultural industry is why the picture of a modern-day farmer no longer shows a tractor driving near a big red barn and a silo, an image often brought to mind at the mention of farmers. A more realistic depiction of today's farmer, however, is quite different: It shows an individual in a biohazard suit, looking a little more like Walter White from the later seasons of *Breaking Bad*.

Chemicals commonly used in modern agriculture include pesticides, insecticides, herbicides, fungicides, and synthetic fertilizers. Farmers spray their land, crops, and even animals with variations of these chemicals, depending on occasion and application. Pesticides created to hold off weeds or insects often have one of two negative effects: They either kill off pieces of the area's natural ecosystem, or the pests they are generated to kill develop a resistance and come back twice as strong as previously. The latter results in an even more toxic substitute being used in following years. US farmers use more than 750 million pounds of agricultural chemicals each year, of 20,000 varieties.[112] Many of these chemicals are used in such excess that the ground cannot absorb them. Runoff, usually carried by rain, begins to spread into nearby waterways and ecosystems. Not only is the farm itself affected, but everything connected to it (including neighbors who are downhill) suffers as well.

Residue from chemicals ends up on our produce and on the crops fed to food animals. Food animals ingest these chemicals, diminishing their health (and quality of life), resulting in a lower-quality food product. This problem surfaces on all levels of food production. The Food Empowerment Project recently released an article that summed this issue up best:

> The residues of these chemicals are found at every level of the food chain, and—through the process of bioaccumulation— become more concentrated the higher up the chain one looks. Meaning, in a system that runs the gamut from microorganisms to humans, people who eat animal products get the highest dosage of toxins.[113]

Farms raising food animals have an issue to face as well. The excess runoff manure pollutes streams and waterways. This adds to the existing problem of fertilizer runoff, which affects the surrounding wildlife and ecosystems. Groundwater infected with nitrites cannot sustain a healthy ecosystem, and often causes the death of the fish in those streams and waterways. "Factory farm runoff also causes algal blooms that kill fish by depleting water of its oxygen, contributing to the formation of hundreds of 'dead zones' worldwide where sea creatures cannot survive."[114]

Pollution due to our modern farming systems and the chemicals used is everyone's problem.

8

America's Most Wanted... Ingredients

(*Research Note*: Information in this chapter is a compilation of research derived from the following sources: Work written by Andrea Donsky of Naturally Savvy Online, particularly the article entitled "7 Scary Food Additives to Avoid;"[115] many works by Joseph Mercola, most specifically his article named "7 Worst Ingredients in Food;"[116] Vivian Goldschmidt, MA, who wrote "12 Dangerous and Hidden Food Ingredients in Seemingly Healthy Foods;"[117] Cat Perry of *Men's Fitness Online*, who wrote "The 9 Scariest Food Additives You're Eating Right Now;"[118] and the alarmingly enlightening book by Russell L. Blaylock: *Excitotoxins: The Taste That Kills.*[119])

By this time, surely you're aware of the controversy and possible agenda behind the ingredients in our food. Even skeptics can, at the very least, acknowledge that most of our food (for whatever reasons) is extremely unhealthy to consume. We have looked at some of the dangerous ingredients already, but there are others to watch for as well. As we will cover in a later chapter, one good, first step in improving your diet is to begin to remove these ingredients from your plate. You may eliminate them all at once, or you may choose a slower route, adjusting one ingredient at a time. It's important to make sure you put into place a plan that allows for follow-through; it helps to decide that you are adopting a new lifestyle rather than making an "overnight overhaul." Changes that last will take time, and *each step in the right direction is a small success to celebrate*. This list is made as of winter of 2017, and it will be up to the reader to be vigilant on their own behalf in watching for aliases. As the market shifts and buyers become wary, labeling *will* change, new ingredient aliases and other marketing "tricks" *will* update as well. As stated earlier, "buyer beware."

High-Fructose Corn Syrup (HFCS)

High-fructose corn syrup is extremely dangerous because it can only be processed by the liver, which makes it more similar to alcohol than regular sugar. Because of this, unlike regular sugar, which at least has the potential to be regulated into energy, it is directly converted into fat. The heavy load HFCS places on the liver causes liver damage and directly contributes to obesity, obesity-related disorders, insulin resistance, increased belly fat, heart disease, liver disfunction, hyperactivity, chronic illness, and the feeding frenzy that it sends cancer cells on. It is often a GMO product, which adds to the risk.

This product is made from yellow dent corn, and has been shown to increase belly fat and insulin resistance. It has *also* been directly linked to a particularly long list of chronic diseases such as liver failure or heart disease. Because cancer cells metastasize differently in the presence of HFCS than with other sugars, this is the deadliest form of sugar in relation to cancer risk.

Particularly used in beverages, this ingredient is found in many unexpected food items. Why is it used? Because it is inexpensive. When an overabundance of corn flooded the market, the corn industry was compromised. The answer was to subsidize the production, allowing crops to be sold at low rates. This subsidization allows HFCS to be one of the cheapest forms of sweetener available. The danger is increased by the way it "sneaks" into your daily diet via pathways of unsuspected carriers like salad dressing, crackers, fruit products, and even medications. Many manufacturers have tried to claim that it is no different than regular sugar, but this is an all-out lie. Dr. Joseph Mercola explains:

High–fructose corn syrup contains free-form monosaccharides of fructose and glucose, it cannot be considered biologically equivalent to sucrose (sugar), which has a glycosidic bond that links the fructose and glucose together, and which slows its breakdown in the body. Fructose is primarily metabolized by your liver, because your liver is the only organ that has the transporter for it. Since all fructose gets shuttled to your liver, and, if you eat a typical Western-style diet, you consume high amounts of it, fructose ends up taxing and damaging your liver in the same way alcohol and other toxins do. And just like alcohol, fructose is metabolized directly into fat…which leads to mitochondrial malfunction, obesity and obesity-related diseases.[120]

Dr. Mercola recommends avoiding the ingredient altogether, but if consumption is unavoidable, he advises keeping intake below 25 grams per day.

Synthetic Trans Fats

Trans fats are made when vegetable oils are hydrogenated, which is a process that changes them from liquid to solid fat. They are often listed as "partially hydrogenated oils" or "hydrogenated oils" on food labels. Trans fats increase the length of time that foods can remain on a shelf before the expiration date and they also stabilize flavor. Trans fats have been linked to cancer, diabetes, decreased immune function, reproduction issues, cellular deterioration, heart disease, and inflammation of the joints. The body's triglyceride level elevates when this is present. LDLs (bad cholesterol) rise and HDLs (good cholesterol) drop under the influence of this ingredient, causing the body to have twice as much difficulty absorbing this fat as it does saturated fats. This increases risk of heart attack and has been linked to both breast cancer and prostate cancer. Trans fats hinder the body's cancer-fighting agents, impede with the body's ability to properly process insulin, reduce the effectiveness of the immune system, and cause fertility issues.[121] Other connections lead to Alzheimer's disease, diabetes—and, of course, our dear old friend that starts it all, obesity.

To avoid trans fats, we must watch labels cautiously. Because the FDA allows manufacturers to claim "zero trans fat" on products containing less than .5 grams per serving, we must be certain the serving size is accurate. For example, if a food product comes individually prepackaged, presumably to be consumed in one sitting, then we would presume the serving size on the nutrition label will state that the entire package is equivalent to one serving. However, if the food item contains between .5–1.0 gram of trans fat, then the manufacturer is allowed to state on the nutrition label that one serving size equals half the package. The nutrition label says that the number of servings contained in the package is *two*, not *one*. Because the food was divided in half to calculate the "serving size," the amount of trans fat would drop to below .5 gram "per serving." This makes the product eligible for the trans fat reading to be "0." The manufacturer can then advertise on the front of the package, "Zero Trans Fats!" If you eat several servings of these types of food items in a day—such as a meal replacement bar or a similar snack you would eat on the go—you could take in several grams of trans fats over the course of that day, all the while assuming that you are taking in none because of its "Zero Trans Fat!" label.

Other names that might mean your trans fat is hiding within include partially hydrogenated oils, hydrogenated oils, DATEM, monoglycerides and diglycerides. Other oils that say "hydrogenated" may be labeled separately as well, such as hydrogenated cottonseed oil.

Oils that state "fully hydrogenated" are not considered trans fats.

Monosodium Glutamate (MSG)

MSG has been covered in this book as an excitotoxin, but as a specific ingredient, it has other woes the reader should be wary of as well.

MSG is an artificial flavor enhancer found in many foods these days, from fast food to processed food and other shelf-stable items at your local grocery store. It has been deemed generally safe by the FDA, but has been known to be unsafe for approximately seventy years. Some of the frightening symptoms are facial numbness, heart palpitations, nausea, weakness, swelling, migraines, seizures, headaches, hives or other allergic reactions, muscle tightness, fatigue, and a tingling or burning sensation in the mouth, head, and neck. It interferes with temperature control, pain regulation, and sleep habits, as well as with the function of the heart, gastrointestinal tract, lungs, and even the bladder.

MSG is also linked to obesity, type 2 diabetes, metabolic syndrome, Lou Gehrig's disease, Parkinson's disease, and other issues that involve the brain. It also overstimulates the nervous system. Over time, the stimulation begins to "stack up," heightening the response to MSG. This means that an allergy or reaction may seem small or even go unnoticed until the underlying issue gets out of hand. This slow escalation in symptoms allows an ambiguity that prevents identifying MSG as the cause of these issues. Studies have shown that MSG is particularly dangerous to pregnant or nursing mothers and their babies, because infants and young children are *four times* more sensitive to MSG than adults. Because of this, the substance has also been linked to learning disabilities, addiction risk, and behavioral and emotional problems, especially in those who were exposed as infants.

Because at times glutamic acid is otherwise a common neurotransmitter in the brain (MSG is about 78 percent glutamic acid, which the brain uses to initiate functions within the body related to the eyes, pancreas, brain, nervous system, and other organs for certain functions within the body), MSG can more intrusively interfere with brain chemistry. This means that while we don't always suffer the consequences immediately, the brain is *extremely* vulnerable to destruction caused by this ingredient. MSG affects the pituitary and adrenal glands, thyroid, ovaries, testes, and pancreas. It causes radical hormone fluctuations, contributing to hormone imbalance (which contributes to obesity and disrupts emotions), and even causes mood swings. Other side effects include impaired memory perception, cognition, and motor issues.

We pay a great price for our ingestion of MSG. So why are we using it? Because it stabilizes and enhances the flavor of what we're eating, generally making us want to *eat more* of that product. Recall that this ingredient is a *stimulant*, and because of this, we *feel* excited about the taste (remember, this is how the word "excitotoxin" originated).[122] But, why is MSG generally recognized as safe (GRAS) by the FDA? Partly because these adverse reactions stack up over time. Because they don't manifest immediately, the MSG is allowed to hide within the shadow of doubt. But, behind the scenes, excitatory neurotransmitters are working through the brain, as we discussed before, firing rapid signals and permanently destroying cells.

This ingredient is quite the shapeshifter, going unnoticed in our food because of its many pseudonyms, some of which are autolyzed yeast extract, yeast extract, autolyzed yeast, hydrolyzed vegetable protein, vegetable powder, maltodextrin, sodium caseinate, and even citric acid. There are nearly fifty forms of MSG (at this time), and as consumers get wiser, it appears with more new names. This ingredient is found in nearly all prepackaged foods, premade foods, and fast foods. Hot dogs, sausages, soups, salad dressing, many vegetarian foods, diet beverages, and more contain this ingredient under one name or another. This is one of the hardest ingredients to eliminate from our diets because of its ambiguity. However, diligent and vigilant consumers eventually learn what names to look for, and they become successful at removing them from their diet.

Artificial Colors

Just since 1990, the use of artificial colors in food has increased by 50 percent. It's alarming to know that more than fifteen million pounds of artificial food dye gets pumped into US-produced foods each year. Cereals, cookies, fruit products, candy, and even pharmaceutical drugs are only a handful of the myriad products that include these ingredients. Despite the revolution to create more natural food and the increasing growth of "healthy" and "organic" markets, appearance and instant gratification still lure in many consumers.

This *could* be because many are still unaware of the dangers of these carcinogens. You read that correctly: They are carcinogens, or cancer-causing agents. Many food dyes are petroleum-derived. Because "artificial colors" is a blanket phrase that covers many similar ingredients, I will not list the dangers of each ingredient, but I will list a few. For example, Red #3 has been linked to chromosomal damage and thyroid tumors, Red # 40 has spurred lymph tumors in lab testing, and Yellows #5 and #6 have been linked to thyroid and kidney tumors, lymphocytic lymphomas, and chromosomal damage.[123]

The belief that food dyes are associated with hyperactivity, attention deficit disorder, and hyperactivity within children is certainly not to be ignored. It is no secret that even children *without* behavioral disorders respond negatively to excessive amounts of artificial coloring in their diets. In the European Union, foods containing these dyes are required to feature warning labels that state the products "may have an adverse effect on activity and attention in children."[124] Yet in America, these dyes are commonly found in products marketed *specifically* to children! Behavioral problems aren't the only issues linked to these food dyes, although they are probably the most common complaint. Allergies and cancer are also among the list of ailments linked to food color. Yellow #5 "may not only be contaminated with several cancer-causing chemicals, but it's also linked to hyperactivity, hypersensitivity and other behavioral effects in children."[125]

Diligent shoppers can find other options. Some synthetic dyes have been banned from use in American food, which is encouraging. Other natural substances like beta-carotene and carmine are less damaging, but avoiding added color altogether is the safest bet.

So, why are we using these ingredients? We see a familiar theme again: because food is marketed to the consumer's sense of excitement and thrill. Recall as well that these ingredients are often included in foods packaged in containers featuring popular cartoon characters or adventurous scenes geared toward kids. These "hyped-up" products are being marketed to our children in place of other entertainment. (Just a side note: If we would turn off the TV and encourage our kids to get outside and play, or to use their own creativity through activities or crafts, they won't need to find so much "excitement" in their food. This could be the topic of another entire book, so I'll be brief: We might be forcing a sedentary lifestyle on our children and then subsidizing the missing excitement with food. This is a double whammy and a double injustice we are serving our children!)

Artificial Sweeteners

In light of recent studies revealing the dangers of sugar, many people are supplementing their diets with artificial sweeteners. Sadly, what they don't realize is that these are even worse than real sugar. Because many artificial sweeteners are excitotoxins or they stimulate in a similar fashion to excitotoxins, they create an overstimulation with an identical or similar effect on the brain. For example, the amino acids found in aspartame attack the body's cells, including brain cells, causing overstimulation and damage almost identical to that caused by other excitotoxins. Because artificial sweeteners throw digestive enzymes out of balance and alter gut-barrier function, inflammatory bowel disease is one of the least threatening conditions the digestive system faces with the introduction of these chemicals.

Many studies have linked artificial sweeteners to weight gain, imbalance in the gut flora, which is the beneficial bacteria found in the gut that helps aid healthy digestion (an *essential* element that we'll discuss in an upcoming chapter), headaches, dizziness, mood changes, convulsions, rashes, memory loss, and even leukemia. Aspartame has been associated with sleep disorders, seizures, headaches, and neurological effects as well.

Artificial sweeteners are another ingredient that hides in many products. Aside from finding them in foods, they're also used to replace sugar in children's medicines. The logic behind that is somewhat understandable, but it is simply deleting one dangerous ingredient and replacing it with another that is even worse.

Sodium Nitrite and Sodium Nitrate

Sodium nitrite and sodium nitrate, when used as ingredients in our food, cause side effects such as dizziness, headaches, nausea, and vomiting. Nitrates combine with stomach acids to produce nitrosamines, an element leading to cancers associated with the pancreas, colon, rectum, stomach, brain, esophagus, bladder, and oral areas.

These ingredients have also been related to health issues such as allergies and neurological disorders. They can be used either as colorants, or to preserve prefabricated meat selections such as bacon, hotdogs, sausage, and lunch meats.

Why are we using this ingredient? Because many of the products they're used in (such as hot dogs, lunch meats, even your holiday ham!) are sold in the refrigerator section; they're not frozen to prevent waste. For food manufacturers to make as much money as possible, it is necessary to extend the shelf-life of these products. This makes sense; after all, it's prudent to try not to waste anything and a business must look out for its bottom line. But it should not do so at the cost of the consumer's well-being.

An increasing selection of lunch meats, hotdogs, and other items are available that do not have added sodium nitrites/nitrates. These may cost a little more, and (as of now) they can be a little harder to find. However, don't be fooled by "all-natural" labeling on some of these products. Flip them over and read the ingredient list on the back. Many labeled "all-natural" still have nitrite added.

Artificial Flavors

"Artificial flavors" is a blanket phrase used to describe synthetic ingredients that are made to taste like the food you think you're eating. These ingredients, by their very nature, warrant one response: *gross*! They're simply designed to trick your taste buds into believing that you are eating a certain kind of food when in fact, you are eating something different.

Aside from the factor of disgust, there is an additional problem with the labeling associated with these elements: The singular name "artificial flavor" can indicate that there is *one* synthetic ingredient included for flavoring, but most often it indicates that a *blend* of artificial components has been added to create a flavor. One example of this is "strawberry flavor," which is a conglomeration of *forty-nine man-made chemical ingredients*.[126] The most commonly used artificial "butter flavor" (containing diacetyl, a chemical linked to Alzheimer's disease and other issues involving the interruption of brain health) is made of over one hundred synthetic chemicals.[127]

Because this all-inclusive name hides many other ingredients, it can also include genetically engineered flavor enhancers. The danger with this is if you buy something that includes "strawberry flavor," you can't be certain exactly *what* chemicals you are eating, or how many *different* ones you are eating. As long as the chemicals going into each of these flavorings have been categorized as "generally recognized as safe (GRAS)" by the FDA, then food manufacturers aren't required to itemize each ingredient within these "artificial flavors." This is done to protect "proprietary formulas" belonging to the companies that produce the products.

What does this mean? The producers don't want to give away their recipes by listing their "secret" ingredients! Under the heading of "trade secrets," artificial flavors provide a back door through which many chemicals are allowed to sneak into your food in a perfectly legal way for "the protection of the food manufacturer."

Also frightening about such labels is that they make it nearly impossible to identify a food allergy or prevent allergic reactions. The very premise of such a label should have no place on our food. When we allow this type of ingredient and its labeling to continue, we are essentially saying that we are content to things made of toxic chemicals that *pose as a certain food*, so long as they add enough chemical content to the final product that that our brains are tricked into believing that it's the food we think it is.

Butylated Hydroxyanisole (BHA), Butylated Hydrozytoluene (BHT), and Tertiary Butylhydroquinone (TBHQ)

Like so many of our other friends on this ingredients list, these preservatives increase the shelf life of prefabricated foods. These have been linked to health issues including but not limited to allergies, neurological disorders, and cancer. BHA and BHT have a negative effect on kidney and liver function, and petroleum-based TBHQ has been associated with nausea, vomiting, tinnitus, and cancer. (TBHQ is so deadly that just 5 grams of it can kill you![128]) These chemicals have been shown to be carcinogenic by the Department of Health and Human Services.[129]

Propyl gallate, an antioxidant preservative to keep fats and oils from going rancid, is often used in conjunction with BHA and BHT. It is found in a wide variety of products, ranging from cosmetics to cooking oils, chips, broths, meat products, and even chewing gums. It is also inconclusively linked to cancer, although this study is new and still under development.

Sodium Benzoate and Benzoic Acid

These preservatives are added to acidic foods to keep microorganisms from growing within them. The problem with these seems minor until sodium benzoate is introduced to ascorbic acid (vitamin C), forming benzene, which is a chemical that causes leukemia and other cancers. This has also been linked to allergic reactions as well.

Potassium Bromate

A preservative used in breads and baked goods to help develop a fluffy and voluminous consistency, this ingredient is used less often these days, as it has been banned in every industrialized country other than the US and Japan. Many companies now opt for a safer alternative, but do continue to keep an eye out for this ingredient, including watching for it under other names.

Sulfites

Found in dried fruit, flavored vinegar, sausages, wines, and other foods, sulfites' biggest mark against them is that they can be dramatic allergens. They are linked to allergy-induced headaches, bowel irritability, behavioral problems, and rashes. The biggest risk with allergies related to sulfites is that airways become constricted rapidly among asthmatics.

Other Preservatives

By now, it is safe to conclude that all synthetic preservatives are harmful on one level or another. The body simply does not know how to recognize and process man-made chemicals. For example, polysorbates 60, 65, and 80 have been linked to severe anaphylactic shock and infertility. Potassium sorbate has been associated with DNA damage. The list continues for what could become an extensive set of research volumes. Many of the chemicals in our food products in America are *banned* in other countries.

9

No Guts, No Glory

At this point, I'm certain that you're now aware of the many reasons our modern American diet needs to change, so now we'll begin to cover the transition into what you can do next to begin this change. At this pivotal moment in the book, I want to remind the reader of my own story. After my surgery, which was successful from a traditional, *medical* standpoint, I continued to suffer from excruciating pain. Test after test revealed that I was healing tremendously by the doctor's standards, but the source of the pain remained a mystery. However, the more I began to dig for answers within the holistic realm, I started to see people making connections between their own previously ambiguous, almost disconnected symptoms. These people were, with the help of holistic doctors, drawing a line between these symptoms to a root source, like some invisible connect-the-dots puzzle within their bodies—and they were finding true relief.

After pursuing treatment with a holistic doctor, I finally, *finally* was given a central diagnosis that explained the varying symptoms I had suffered all of those years. As I said in the first chapter, I learned that the core issue was Leaky Gut Syndrome. You may be thinking at this point, "My gut feels fine. That's not my problem," but before you put the book down, humor me by reading this chapter. I will list the symptoms of this very common condition—some you might recognize in your own life—that affects people all across our country today. Recall that in my story, this *one core issue* was the hub at which my entire life was constantly interrupted by this undiagnosed chronic illness. I would wager that many are manifesting this very illness, but are unaware, because this syndrome is not recognized within our modern, Western, traditional medical conventions.

Before going any farther, I also must recommend that you get a good holistic doctor to help you customize a health plan suited to your needs. Some of the information in this chapter will be specific to my case. If you have been seeing a medical doctor, it's very important that you *do not* discontinue that treatment until you have found a holistic replacement for it. Consult a holistic doctor in person, so he or she can conduct a physical examination and be made aware of all of your circumstances in order to customize a treatment plan *for your needs*.

Some of what you read in this book may not be endorsed by a traditional medical doctor. Holistic practices fall outside the scope of much Western medical training. It is knowledge lost. Recall that when I was heading into surgery, Katherine asked the doctor if probiotics would help me, and he answered that there was "no science to back that idea." This is not to villainize the surgeon who worked on me. On the contrary, I could not have asked for a cleaner surgery when it was time to have 16 inches of my colon cut out. But medical doctors are working within the realms of their medical school training, which largely involves pharmaceutically treating symptoms that have *already manifested.* Traditional doctors often aren't even given the opportunity to act in a preventative way, as most people don't go to doctors until they're sick. On top of this, their hands are often tied because they're restricted by FDA regulations. The FDA endorses treatments that are primarily pharmaceutical, many traditional doctors are restricted to what they are *able* to recommend. Further, because our society is filled with so many people who live on the border of being sick, many of the numbers that come back on lab results fall within "normal" ranges, when they *should* be cause for concern.

I say this so you will understand that if you take this book to a medical doctor, he or she will probably agree that eliminating toxic ingredients from your diet "can't hurt," but the physician might not stress how important it is for you to make these lifestyle changes. I can tell you from personal experience (as verified by the three natural medicines doctors named at the end of this book whose practices and advice literally saved my life) that the holistic approach is what finally cured my ailments, healed my organs, and restored my energy and well-being.

And I'm not making this important point just because I feel better. Along the way, my dramatic health improvement has been verified through real science.

For example, when I first met Dr. Joshua Vance, he ran a series of tests on me to see where my cortisone, adrenals, hormone and organ functions were registering. One test in particular—a full health screening, including a panel of bloodwork, which examined, among other things, vitamins, minerals, liver, thyroid function, and cholesterol—illustrated that my liver was under enormous duress due to a fatty-liver enzyme count of 183 (which can lead to all sorts of liver complications, liver disease, and, if not addressed, ultimately liver failure—not to mention tremendous strain to the immune system, since liver function is key to overall health). My thyroid was showing signs of stress and hyperactivity, I was borderline hypoglycemic, and on my way to becoming diabetic, my bad cholesterol was severely high, increasing my risk of cardiovascular disease and heart attack. The test confirmed, as stated previously, that my testosterone was really low, at four times lower than the average for a male my age, according to hormone specialists I had seen previously. I was at stage 3 adrenal burnout (Leaky Gut Syndrome had stripped my body of all natural forms of energy and I was functioning on adrenals that barely got me through each day), and I was completely devoid of several vitamins I needed to function (most Americans are severely vitamin deficient, because modern foods no longer provide essential vitamins in adequate amounts).

But several months after starting a regiment of supplementation, an improved diet, and lifestyle changes, a whole string of tests was run again. I was elated to learn that my fatty liver tissue had dropped from 183 to 29 (traditional doctors are satisfied with reading under 150, so this was an astronomical drop)! I was nowhere near becoming a diabetic, my testosterone count had come up dramatically, and I had my levels of all the obscure but essential vitamins and minerals like E, K, A, B, and magnesium were good. My adrenals had dramatically recovered, my thyroid and hormone health had improved to "better than the healthy average" for men my age, my white blood cell count had become optimal-strong, my blood lipids showed that my cholesterol was in the ideal-healthy range, and my saturated animal fats were nonexistent. In short, these improvements mean my body responded to the lifestyle adjustments and was able to begin repairing itself to reverse the damage to my liver and immune system and to finally bring me back to a sustainable condition for avoiding the onslaught of disease.

Having said that, let me back up and add a few more critical details. The longer my recovery from surgery continued without relief from most of the symptoms I had been experiencing, the more I realized that another issue had gone unaddressed. I was surprised once I started connecting all the puzzle pieces and began to realize how far back in time the issue had started. After meeting a few different holistic doctors and finding one I felt good about working with, we began to customize a health plan for me. Because my core issue, Leaky Gut Syndrome, had gone untreated for so long, it had escalated into many other health problems that I dealt with over the years. It had caused inflammation throughout my system and had caused the other issues that I discussed in the first chapter of this book. I had even escalated to a diagnosis of stage III adrenal fatigue (I was quickly progressing to the fourth and final stage of adrenal fatigue, a side effect of leaky gut, wherein a patient becomes bedridden and can develop heart disease and many other life-threatening conditions quickly). When I began to address the source problem, I finally began to feel relief from all the other symptoms that had interrupted my quality of life for years.

Ironically, after all my searching for a diagnosis, and then eventually during my hunt for a good holistic doctor, my quest led me back to a resource I had access to all along: the friend and chiropractor I mentioned earlier, Dr. Joshua Vance. I can't say enough about this man and how he has helped me during this lifestyle overhaul. He always weaves biblical principles into my treatment, assures me that I am on the right track, and has let me know that if he ever reaches the end of his knowledge of how to help me (a scenario I seriously doubt), he knows who to bring in for more expertise. His vast knowledge and bedside manner are evidence of his devotion, and his "psychological first aid," as my good friend Mark Taylor calls it, is second to none.

The more I learn about my diagnosis, the more I realize how, for years, I was ignorantly contributing to my own demise. Even my attempts to help myself worsened my situation. Gut flora, which we will talk about in the upcoming pages, is extremely important to our overall health, yet it is one of the most overlooked aspects of Western medical practices. I now know that every round of antibiotics I took—especially that initial ninety-day round—caused mounting damage to the gut flora within my intestines, causing further pain, illness, and immune debilitation. *And,* unlike so many of my doctors had seemed to relay, *diet is crucial to gut flora.*

The gut is now being recognized—mostly by holistic doctors—as the culprit behind hundreds of diseases. Every condition I suffered for years was a spinoff of a sick gut. This is because of toxic diet and improper treatment of chronic illness. So many of these diseases are addressed by medications that deal with *symptoms*, but they don't target the *underlying problem*, which is often the gut. A healthy gut prevents many diseases and fights more effectively diseases that are contracted. When the gut is in good shape, we can avoid having to take unnecessary medications, giving hope beyond the pharmacy. Achieving a healthy gut, for many people, comes through improving diet and lifestyle. Until somebody introduced me to the hope that I could be healed by changing what I was doing to my gut, I was on a path that only led to more chronic illness and possibly more surgeries. I had done the things that people say are wise to do, like lose weight and exercise. I had taken the meds the doctors prescribed, and even had the surgical procedures I had been told would help me. At the end of it all, I was still left with the possibility that I could one day need additional colon surgery, if the diverticulosis were to come back in a different part of my intestines. That is a dark, hopeless road that would have only led to more despair.

The entire time I was searching for healing, the answers were right in front of me, hidden in plain sight. A few key people in my life had mentioned natural healing, but I had refused to listen, stubbornly leaning on modern medicine and thinking that my condition was too advanced to be helped through natural means. I was wrong. What I needed had been there since the beginning, and it goes all the way back to Genesis, when God gave us use of all the vegetation. For centuries, plants and herbs have been mankind's pharmaceuticals. For the modern holistic doctor, this is nothing new. And those who believe themselves to be "finally discovering" the healing that natural means have to offer are only going back to the basics.

Other Symptoms of Leaky Gut Syndrome

Many people don't realize that autoimmune diseases are formed as a result of Leaky Gut Syndrome. This means if you have a problem in your gut, this may not be the area where you are experiencing pain. The symptoms of an unhealthy gut can manifest in dozens of ways—not just in abdominal pain—that can often go untreated because they are difficult to diagnose or simply attributed to aging. If you are suffering from some of these other symptoms, it's possible that you have Leaky Gut Syndrome and are not yet experiencing enough intestinal pain to realize what you're dealing with. Consider some of the symptoms below:[130]

- Constant fatigue, inability to get enough sleep even when you go to bed early. Do you have to consume sugary snacks, soft drinks, or even energy drinks to get through a regular day?
- Surges of depression or anxiety, or the need to stop and "breathe" through stressful (or not-so-stressful) situations
- Constant dehydration
- Hair loss
- Insomnia
- Rapid heartbeat, the sensation that your heart is racing, or waves of panic
- Pre-diabetic symptoms
- Weight gain or loss that seems unexplainable, or "stubborn" fat
- Hormonal imbalances that don't make medical sense or seem unconnected to a source. This could manifest in irregular menstruation, miscarriage, and blood clots in women, or in men, low testosterone (and in my case, low sperm count).
- Numbness or tingling in legs, feet, and hands
- Stomach, abdominal, or intestinal cramping or pain, chronic diarrhea or chronic constipation, or an alternation between the two
- Fatty liver or liver dysfunction
- Abdominal cramping or pain, or feelings that the stomach is becoming more sensitive to foods with age
- The development of food allergies
- Kidney dysfunction
- Heartburn or acid reflux conditions

- Depression, anxiety, Attention Deficit/Hyperactivity Disorder
- Frequent headaches
- Diagnosis of autoimmune conditions such as lupus, chronic fatigue syndrome, Crohn's disease, or adrenal fatigue
- Adult acne, eczema, or psoriasis
- Inflammatory conditions such as tendinitis, arthritis, or symptoms that are labeled, "inflammatory bowel disease," "irritable bowel syndrome," or other inflammation in the intestines

But what is Leaky Gut Syndrome, really? When the gut is not functioning properly, it is unable to break down food. This results in the system transferring particles of this undigested food into the bloodstream for the liver to filter out. As the undigested food particles travel through the bloodstream, the body recognizes these particles as an enemy in the body. The immune system then attacks those particles as an enemy, dealing with them in the same way they would deal with a virus or bacteria that is attacking the body. As the body continues to place this load on the liver, toxins become so backlogged that the body goes into a sort of "panic state," raising its white blood cell count to eradicate the toxins as the immune system continues to work in a hypervigilant state. Over time, the immune system becomes fatigued, and the lines begin to blur between what is an enemy, what is organic to the body, and what is just a misplaced food element. Soon, the body's defense mechanism is to develop an enmity with things it would not normally fight against. This is how food sensitivities (similar to an allergy) are developed, and also how the body begins to attack itself in certain areas (similar to the way the immune system will attack the guts in a person who has Crohn's disease). Over time, the body works so much harder than necessary, both fighting against itself and repairing itself from its own attacks, that disorders like adrenal fatigue and chronic fatigue syndrome develop. Because of its heightened state, the immune system becomes tired, causing frequent sickness. In general, all the systems begin breaking down because nothing is working *properly*, while everything is working *too hard*. This process destroys the body's natural adrenal response to stress or emergencies and leads to more severe exhaustion, causing even more demand on the already-taxed systems.

My Transition into Holistic Therapy

During my period of working out (around 2009), I was doing one of the worst things I could for my body. I didn't realize I was suffering from adrenal fatigue at the time, which meant that all those times I was pushing myself so hard physically to regain health, I was actually burning what little bit of energy my adrenals had been able to stock up, which was creating further disruption of my immune system as well. If I had known then what I know now, I would have realized that three ten-minute, light cardio workouts per week would have been much safer than pushing my body the way I was.

Ironically, the section of colon that was removed was no longer infected with diverticulitis at the time of my surgery. Once removed and inspected, my surgeon revealed that the multiple weeks of antibiotics had successfully killed the infection. But, as I approached the day of surgery, I felt no decrease in the pain, despite the apparent victory over infection. We knew, based on an emergency room CT scan performed the month before, that the initial cause of the pain was, in fact, diverticulitis once again. The removed section did indeed have *diverticulosis* (the polyps that become infected and lead to *diverticulitis*), which meant probable future infections if not removed, but the pain I now suffered, I was told, couldn't still be stemming from the infection. I would learn, in time, that the pain was due to my gut's lack of flora, inflammation, and escalated long-term aggravation within my intestines.

My Leaky Gut Syndrome was hitting an all-time intensification, causing my pain. When the surgery had healed and I was still experiencing agony, I was left with the underlying cause that still needed to be investigated and healed.

In addition to Leaky Gut Syndrome, I soon found out that food sensitivities were creating additional strain on my gut. Dr. Joshua Vance ran an immunoglobulin (IgG) panel on me. This test "measures the level of certain immunoglobulins, or antibodies, in the blood. Antibodies are proteins made by the immune system to fight antigens, such as bacteria, viruses, and toxins."[131] In a nutshell, this test identifies food sensitivities, and it revealed many that were contributing to my Leaky Gut Syndrome. Remember that I said I had traded cereals for yogurts, dairy products, and eggs? It turned out that I have a sensitivity to dairy products; eliminating them from my diet helped relieve my pain. The dietary changes I've made are a lifestyle, and believe me, if I make a mistake and eat something I am sensitive to, I pay a big price. I also discovered that many of the healthy foods and supplements I was taking to improve my health (ginger, quinoa, apples, eggs, and cinnamon) were furthering inflammation and delaying my path to full healing because I am allergic to them.

The Right Tests for the Right Diagnosis

Once you've chosen a holistic doctor, allow him or her to run the tests that will reveal the information necessary to help you. Joshua Vance started his treatment of me with a complete physical exam and a thorough history of my symptoms, including a detailed inventory of my diet. He then ran (as I mentioned) the IgG panel, a stool analysis, a complete blood count (CBC), a complete metabolic panel (CMP), and he performed extensive, broad-spectrum lab work to check for issues with my thyroid, determine whether I had nutritional deficiencies, and examine the possibility of other underlying culprits.

Based on this information, I learned what nutrients I was deficient in so I could begin taking supplements. Dietary supplementation is essential, as we have established in this book that even our best foods are declining in essential nutrients at a rapid pace. Finding a good brand of supplements can be difficult, as many can be expensive, while others aren't easily absorbed into the body. On top of this, supplement brands must be held to the same level of scrutiny and quality standards that we use when choosing which food brands to trust. An example of this is the recently announced purchase of Atrium Innovations, makers of Garden of Life supplements, by Nestle.[132] I personally found this news alarming, because when dealing with a food company that is content to include so many dangerous ingredients in its food products, I am concerned that they might become the power behind the nutritional supplementation of that food as well. Time will tell.

Tests Are Expensive!

The tests your holistic doctor might want to run are prohibitively expensive, but it is important to remember that you cannot heal your gut—or your body—if you don't know what it's up against. Have a stool sample run to determine where your gut chemistry stands currently and where it needs to be. Go over dietary history with your holistic doctor, and establish a plan of action for your diet, even if you are not looking to lose weight. Talk to your holistic doctor about regular dietary supplements and follow through by obtaining and taking them.

An obstacle for some people is that some of these tests aren't covered by traditional medical insurance, leaving us to figure out how we will pay for them out of pocket, which can initially be expensive. In fact, the cost could possibly be a roadblock to opting for the natural pathway. My response is that over the years, I've spent thousands of dollars on conventional medical treatment that, in the end, wasn't the solution to the source of my health problems. Finding out my food sensitivities and how I was nutritionally deficient was a one-time expense that has been life-changing. On top of this, most doctors who are interested in helping you get well will work with you to arrange a monthly payment plan. If your body is dealing with an issue under the surface (and remember, you might not be experiencing gut pain for this to be true; it could be manifesting in any of the ways listed earlier in this chapter) that is possibly escalating, these tests could end up saving you money in the long run—not to mention the pain and unnecessary exposure to harmful medications they could help eliminate. I *highly* recommend following the advice of your holistic doctor and having the necessary tests run, even if it means taking on a payment plan.

That said, if the price of the tests is prohibitive and you decide to do a bit of self-testing to try to identify your food sensitivities, here is a list, taken from Dr. Brownstein's book *Heal Your Leaky Gut*, of common culprits:[133]

- eggs
- fish
- gluten
- dairy
- peanuts
- shellfish
- soy
- tree nuts
- corn
- wheat and other grains with gluten

Below is a list of additional items that could be triggering gastrointestinal distress:

- alcohol
- soda pop or other carbonated or caffeinated drinks, including coffee

- fried or greasy foods
- spicy foods
- excessive sugar
- excessive salt

If you're trying to identify a food sensitivity and for some reason you can't have the IgG panel run, you can try to identify the culprit by eliminating one of the above ingredients for a period of time and watching for any improvement in your symptoms. These changes can take up to three months to register in your body, meaning that it may take eliminating an ingredient for longer than just a few days to notice a difference. Again, I cannot state strongly enough: I recommend discussing this with a holistic doctor and having an IgG panel run rather than trying to find your way through this on your own.

The Importance of Gut Flora

Gut flora, or gut microbiota, is the name for the bacteria living in our intestine. Each person has a unique balance of gut flora that his or her body needs to maintain for good health (this is another reason to consult a holistic doctor: so he or she can personalize a health plan specifically for you). The gut should have over one hundred billion bacteria in it, but chemicals, GMO foods, pesticides, and antibiotics kill some of this and throw the rest off-balance.[134] When these bacteria are not in balance, digestion is interrupted, nutrition is not properly absorbed, and autoimmune responses increase. The intestine is the body's filter, deciding what to discard as waste and to allow into the body. Some bacteria promote disease while others fight it. When the gut flora is out of balance, the filter doesn't work properly. Some say this is merely a genetic predisposition within the gut, but that's not always true. Studies conducted on twins have shown that the gut microbiota was different between the two, one of whom was obese and one of which was not.[135] This means that taking charge of your gut health can change your predisposition toward obesity and disease, and it could possibly even mean that some diseases said to be "hereditary" could be controlled through gut flora as well, as I learned through personal experience.

Certain bacteria associated with disease can produce gas or other chemicals, causing intestinal discomfort.[136] These bacteria are often present in patients diagnosed with irritable bowel syndrome (IBS) and inflammatory bowel disease (IBD), indicating that balance to gut flora can reduce predisposition to or symptoms of these and other digestive conditions.

Healthy gut flora is promoted by a safe, natural diet, with probiotic-rich food, and exercise. Probiotics help restore the balance in gut flora, allowing the gut to properly filter food by expelling waste and fully absorbing the nutrients. Because there is communication between the intestine and the immune system, a balanced gut flora lessens autoimmune responses within the body and overall immune function is optimal. Healthy bacteria within the gut helps balance blood sugar, which minimizes the risk of diabetes and helps keep negative bacteria from adhering to the wall of the gut, resulting in overall better health.[137] Recent studies have also shown that the heart can remain healthier when gut flora is in balance:

> Certain unhealthy species in the gut microbiota may also con-tribute to heart disease by producing trimethylamine N-oxide (TMAO).
>
> TMAO is a chemical that contributes to blocked arteries, which may lead to heart attack or stroke.
>
> Certain bacteria within the microbiome convert choline and L-carnitine, both of which are nutrients found in red meat and other animal-based food sources, to TMAO, potentially increas-ing risk factors for heart disease.[138]

The importance of balance within gut flora impacts many aspects of our health that scientists are only now beginning to connect. That pre-set balance each of our bodies uniquely needs must be found and preserved for each of us to be as healthy as we can be. Recent studies have even shown that healthy gut flora can help cancer patients respond more effectively to treatment:

> Cancer patients with high levels of good gut bacteria appear more likely to respond to immunotherapy, potentially opening up a new way to optimize the use of modern medicines that are highly effective but only work in some people.[139]

Is the Gut the Second Brain?

The health of the gut is even beginning to be connected to our mental health. Because millions of nerves link up the gut and the brain,[140] it is probable that the brain's health is influenced by what's going on in the gut. Dr. Douglas Lord of NAVA Health & Vitality Center reported in 2015:

> The health of your gastrointestinal system is extremely important to your overall well-being. Largely responsible for the critical functions of the body's digestive and immune systems, beneficial bacteria in your digestive system have the capability of affecting your body's vitamin and mineral absorbency, hormone regulation, digestion, vitamin production, immune response, and ability to eliminate toxins, not to mention your overall mental health.[141]

Recent studies are connecting gut flora to such conditions as depression, anxiety, ADHD, and autism. Further, one such investigation showed that people who have Alzheimer's disease exhibit distinct differences in their gut bacteria.

A team of researchers primarily based out of the University of Wisconsin-Madison examined the gut microbiota of twenty-five Alzheimer's patients at the Wisconsin Alzheimer's Disease Research Center and compared their samples with those of twenty-five control subjects matched for age, gender, and health.

Overall, Alzheimer's patients had reduced micro biodiversity, as well as a few noteworthy differences in bacterial abundance.[142]

The study showed a lower level of firmicutes and fiactinobacteria, along with higher levels of bacteroidetes that existed within Alzheimer's patients. "As many as 500 million neurons dwell in the gastrointestinal system and are connected to the brain via the vagus nerve. Thus, gut bacteria have access to the brain via a veritable superhighway and can influence it in both good and bad ways."[143] These agents also affect glucose metabolism, indicating an impact on diabetes and obesity. The study results further connected bacteria within the blood to Parkinson's disease and the body's ability to fight inflammation.

With a better understanding of the importance of gut flora and how the balance in the gut affects the brain, it's no wonder that the gut is becoming known as the second brain. Earlier in the book, we talk about excitotoxins; which are an outright attack on the *first* brain. With a better understanding of how the *second* brain is under attack, it is apparent that our bodies and minds are dealing with a chemical assault that comes from every direction.

Dr. David Brownstein, in his book, *Repair Your Leaky Gut*, suggests that we follow what he calls the four Rs:[144]

Remove: Discontinue eating foods that are toxic, dangerous, allergens, or in any other way distressing to your system.

Replace: Introduce good bacteria to your digestive tract by beginning the habit of adding probiotics.

Reinocculate: Maintain a balance of healthy nutrients, therapies and supplements that promote good gut health and keep inflammation at bay.

Repair: Follow these steps faithfully and allow your gut time to heal.

Grains and Your Gut

As I said in the beginning of the book, despite all my cardio workouts in the year 2009, I never lost the fat off my gut. Some of this increased size, I later realized, was swelling due to inflammation. But this is a common complaint of many people. Those last few pounds want to cling to the same spot on everybody. Why is that? It can be a combination of a couple reasons.

Processed foods can be a huge culprit where stubborn belly fat is concerned. Inflammation has been medically linked to the bulge as well. Because this is the location of your body where these toxins come in, it stands to reason that this is where the inflammation occurs. Contrary to what it may seem, eating the right kinds of fats will help a person shed these extra pounds. When the body is used to living on fatty (the wrong kinds of fats), sugary foods, it finds these cheap, easy calories easier to transfer into energy than the actual process of burning fat. As a result, the body burns sugars and stores fat, eventually burning very little of the incoming fat (this is part of the pre-diabetic condition). Since the average American eats more sugary, high-carbohydrate calories in a day than the body can burn, the results is stubborn fat that the body has nearly forgotten *how* to burn.

In my journey, I was surprised to find that when I cut sugars and fats from my diet, I lost *much* weight, but it wasn't until I eliminated toxic chemicals from my diet and began to take in *enough of the right kind of fats* that I finally began to see this bulge melt away. In my case, this resulted from a combination of reduction in swelling due to alleviated inflammation and actual weight loss due to taking in the right kinds of fat and reminding my body how to burn fat by eating the right foods.

A high level of stress, poor diet, and lack of sleep (the modern theme in nearly every American's life) can also cause a hormone imbalance, which causes belly fat to store and stubbornly hang on for dear life. Carey Rossi of *Health.com* sums it up as follows:

> Tight deadlines, bills, your kids—whatever your source of stress, having too much of it may make it harder for you to drop unwanted pounds, especially from your middle. And it's not just because you tend to reach for high-fat, high-calorie fare when you're stressed, though that's part of it. It's also due to the stress hormone cortisol, which may increase the amount of fat your body clings to and enlarge your fat cells. Higher levels of cortisol have been linked to more visceral fat.... If you are among the 30% of Americans who sleep less than six hours a night, here's one simple way to whittle your waistline: catch more Zs. A 16-year study of almost 70,000 women found that those who slept five hours or less a night were 30% more likely to gain 30 or more pounds than those who slept seven hours. The National Institutes of Health suggest adults sleep seven to eight hours a night.[145]

When I finally identified Leaky Gut Syndrome as my core health problem, and began to make the healthy lifestyle changes necessary to put my health on the right track, as I said before, fat literally melted off my midsection. I've been careful with workouts to avoid demanding more of my adrenals, so very little of my current weight loss is a result of cardio-heavy exercise. The weight loss I have experienced has come from treating my body well, getting enough rest, eating organic foods, supplementing my gut's health, supplementing my diet (which we will discuss in the next chapter), and eliminating foods that I am sensitive to. In doing so, I addressed all of these gut-fat causing culprits. An indirect result was even a reduction of stress, due to eliminated illness.

The Right Diet

I can't outline all the ways you should and should not eat for a healthy gut, because, as we have established, individual food sensitivities, individual gut flora chemistry, and your medical background play a key role in your dietary needs. But once you have identified your food sensitivities, it is important to avoid them. Each time you eat something that interrupts the balance of gut flora, introduces toxins to the system, or aggravates the intestine through allergic reaction, precious progress is being lost and the window for disease opens wider. Ask your holistic doctor what kind of probiotics to take, and follow through. Resist the temptation to "backslide" on any of the changes you need to embrace just because you start feeling better. Remember that those changes are *why* you are feeling better. Avoid toxic chemicals, hormones and pesticides, processed foods, artificial sweeteners (diet soda and colored drinks), as they compromise healthy gut flora and provide fuel for the negative, disease-causing bacteria that work against digestion and wellness. Eat as much organic food as possible. Not only will this preserve gut flora, but it will protect the rest of your body from the effects of these dangerous chemicals we've already covered. Try to avoid antibiotics if possible; if you must take them, talk to your holistic doctor about how to adjust the probiotics you are taking accordingly. (However, a holistic doctor will almost certainly offer an effective natural alternative to anything pharmaceutical. That natural option will still provide healing, but without compromising your body's recovery systems.)

The Importance of Supplements

Besides regular dietary supplements, which will be covered in the next chapter, many steps can be taken to nurture the gut back to health. Some are listed below, but it is important to consult with your holistic doctor for an all-inclusive list of what would be wise for you to use:

- Aloe vera juice—Made from the leaves of the aloe vera plant, this renders a variety of health benefits, including intestinal regularity and liver health.
- Bone broth—Made from animal bones, this contains vital healing elements such as collagen and proline and heals intestinal lining.
- Psyllium husk—This type of organic fiber derived from plant matter is used to regulate the bowel.
- Probiotics—This is good bacteria that helps stabilize and support healthy gut function.
- Turmeric—This is an herb is used as a natural anti-inflammatory.
- Curcumin—This is an herb is used as a natural anti-inflammatory and natural antioxidant.
- Kale—This leafy, green vegetable is known for its status as a "superfood." Kale is good for many health issues, including pain relief, protection against colon-related cancers, and it has an extremely high nutrient content.
- Ginger—This root is grown for its medicinal uses and food flavor; it is good for healing inflammation, reversing disease, and settling the digestive system.
- Green tea—A tea leaf used for its qualities as an antioxidant, green tea features cancer-fighting agents, improves brain function, and even promotes weight loss.
- Pancreatic enzymes—These agents help aid digestion and balance stomach acid.

- Organic fiber—This supplement helps achieve and maintain regularity and keeps the digestive system in balance.
- Bovine colostrum—This milky liquid procured within the first few days after a cow gives birth is rich in proteins, vitamins, minerals, and other disease-combating agents.
- Oregano oil—This oil is derived from the herb oregano, and has antiviral, antifungal, and antibiotic properties.
- Antioxidants—Often found in fresh fruits, these agents protect the body from harmful molecules.
- Apple cider vinegar—This natural liquid serves myriad healthy purposes, including weight-loss support, regulation of cholesterol, gut health support, and blood sugar regulation.
- Flaxseed oil—Derived from flaxseed, this element helps prevent and fight disease while supplying healthy omega-3s.
- Licorice root—This relieves digestive irritation and helps heal stomach ulcers, along with providing many other health benefits, such as being a safe, natural cough expectorant.
- Collagen powder—This great source of healthy amino acids supports digestive health.
- Problotic—These are rich, fermented foods and drinks, such as sauerkraut and kombucha tea.

Find a Good Holistic Doctor

When I decided to proceed with holistic treatment, I did a Google search for holistic doctors and made an appointment with one who seemed qualified and had good reviews online. When I arrived at her office, I immediately found it to be a different experience than visiting traditional medical doctors' offices. Essential oils were being diffused, calming music was being played, and, unlike at a traditional doctor's office, pharmaceutical posters weren't all over the walls. The holistic doctor calmly listened to a lot of my symptoms and my story as I tried to bring her up to speed as much as possible about my fifteen-year journey. She quickly indicated that she recognized my symptoms and could help me establish a plan to leave behind this painful chapter of my life. She assured me there was hope. She told me I would have a new lease on life.

For the first time in a very long time, I left the doctor's office with true hope. For so many years, I had wanted to change my health, and there was a professional who seemed to be able to connect the dots preparing to work with me. This euphoric level of hope made me realize how much anxiety my medical problems had been creating for me over the years. Sometimes it's not until you get a little bit of relief that you realize how much pain or duress you've been in.

The doctor gave me a plan for a detox diet, which I began immediately. Up to this point, I would have said that I had already cleaned up my diet. But after reading the information she gave me, I realized my "healthy" diet still included of all kinds of detrimental ingredients. For example, my "healthier" coffee creamer was still loaded with chemicals. Other simple, easily overlooked culprits in my kitchen were quickly brought to light. With this new information in hand, Katherine and I began to clean house in a whole new way. We threw away nearly anything with chemicals in it—even hygienic products such as toothpaste and deodorant, replacing them with natural options.

For about the first five days of this detox process, I thought I was dying. My body was in a state of withdrawal from all the chemicals it was still used to, even despite my prior efforts at keeping a more natural diet. I experienced terrible headaches, severe nausea, chills, dizziness, intense weakness, and *huge* cravings for anything with carbs, particularly buttered wheat bread (even though I had been eating the organic, expensive bread up to this point). The holistic doctor had scheduled a follow-up appointment for two weeks after our first appointment, but I found myself wondering I could make it that long. I called my friend Mark Taylor again, and he told me that it was detox sickness.

Like an addict experiences?

Yes.

I went through the detox sickness for several days and completed the detox diet, and spent quite some time on the GAPS (gut and psychology syndrome) diet. I *strongly* encourage anyone with any sort of autoimmune disease or chronic digestive condition to research this diet! Later, with the help of another holistic doctor I eventually began working with, I modified the ketone diet (in which a person consumes high amounts of healthy fats, adequate quantities of proteins, and low levels of carbs) to suit my own needs and became pescatarian (vegetarian with the allowance of seafood), which has been an enormous step in healing my gut and my body as a whole. I supplement religiously, using many of the gut supplements listed previously in this chapter, and I also enhance my diet with vitamins and nutrients that my diet may not be providing. I stick to organic foods, buying locally any time possible. My family buys bulk ingredients and we make nearly all our meals from scratch, a topic that will be discussed in the upcoming pages.

But my story with the first holistic doctor I found on Google doesn't end there. I want to share the rest of my experience with the first holistic doctor I worked with. It didn't have the ending one might anticipate. While some of her initial information set me on the right track, follow-up visits did not go well. On my second appointment with her, she found out that I have had a CT scan. Her response was to throw her arms in the air, saying "You're more likely to have cancer now because you had a CT scan!" That comment scared me. It seemed like every time I told her about a chemical I had run across in my food or a medical procedure I had, she found another reason to tell me I had subjected myself to certain doom. By having surgery, I had done irreparable damage to my body by allowing vital organs to be cut out. While admitting there might have been some technical merit to the procedures that I had undergone, her initial responses were always things like, "You let that doctor do what to you?! Oh, that's *criminal!*"

After a comment like this, she would shake her head and click her tongue, making notes in my chart.

One day, she misread the note she had made on my chart about my following appointment. When I commented that I had a different date in my phone's calendar, she said "Oh, your brain fog is really bad! Whoever did your surgery really screwed up!" After a moment of comparing notes, she realized the mistake was hers, but not before she had incited doubt, fear, and insecurity about my recovery in my mind.

Interactions like this continued during my relationship with this doctor. It seemed like every visit or phone call was met with one or two questions answered and three or four new, more frightening questions raised. Every communication I shared with her left me feeling even more anxious than before.

When I talked to my friend Mark Taylor about it, he laughed and said, "Man, you gotta find yourself someone with some good psychological first aid. When I worked at the fire department, we didn't show up at a scene where someone had been shot and yell 'Whoa, you're gonna die!' You tell the patient that it's gonna be okay, tell them what you *are* going to do for them and what they can expect to *happen next*. You don't just tell them how awful this thing that just happened is!"

Later I was telling my sister, Allie, about the situation. Allie was frustrated because she had seen me go through so much over the years, and now that I was so close to true healing, I wasn't even able to enjoy it. She laughingly rolled her eyes and said, "What is she, some kind of nature snob?"

The problem persisted. The closer I got to really good, helpful information, the more fear I was also developing about things I had done in the past that could not be changed. I didn't need to know how I had already damaged my body, I was *well* aware of that. What I needed was information about how to move forward and *heal*. It seemed like I was trading one type of anxiety for another.

One day, Katherine was nearby, listening to my end of a phone call with this doctor. I was asking the doctor if she thought it would be wise for me to have a follow-up colonoscopy to rule out any leftover diverticulosis. (This was before my colonoscopy in 2017.) Her answer was, "If they do another colonoscopy, they're probably going to find more polyps. Truthfully, they'll probably even find cancer. To be honest with you, everybody's got some kind of cancer. If they go looking for it, they'll find it. But what I believe I have outlined for you is a way that you shouldn't have to worry about it regardless. Stay on the diet I have given you, and I'll see you at your next appointment, ok?"

After this phone call, Katherine had enough. She put her foot down.

"This doctor is not good for you. Instead of telling you how to fix the problem, she's just loading you up with more reasons to be anxious and depressed and worried. You're not to see her again."

And I didn't.

Initially, I didn't know what good it would do to include this part of my story in this book, so I intended to skip it. But it is important for a person visiting a holistic doctor for the first time to understand that, like in any other profession, some out there are simply "not a good fit." Many doctors in the natural healing realm are there because they want to see people healed and they are working toward that cause; but like in any other industry, some use their careers as a pedestal to sit on in judgment of others below for subjecting their bodies to medical proce-dures or hazardous, toxic chemicals. Doctors who have this attitude will neither help nor heal you. If you have a similar experience, don't get dis-couraged and give up. Find another doctor and keep trying. My health at the time was so bad that I didn't have a choice but to keep pursuing this avenue. But if I had been given a choice or was pursuing holistic health for less urgent reasons, my experience with this doctor might have been enough to turn me off of the natural healing method forever. I'm sharing this experience with you to encourage you to keep trying. As my sister put it, some "nature snobs" out there will browbeat you with your past, which might include medication, chemicals, or surgery. If you have (and if you're reading this book, the odds are you have done at least one of these things), there is nothing you can do about it now. Beating yourself up (or worse, allowing a medical professional to) over what's in the past will do you absolutely no good. Finding someone who will help you move forward from *here* is essential for your future healing and success.

I can't emphasize this enough: There is a lot of hope for people who are suffering from myriad health problems that Western medical practitioners have conditioned them to accept. I have friends diagnosed with diseases such as Lupus and multiple sclerosis who have put their illnesses into remission through natural healing methods, lifestyle changes, and diet improvements and are for the first time in decades no longer taking pharmaceutical medications.

But it doesn't end here: Throughout my own journey of holistic healing, my eyes were opened to the vast array of treatments that exist via natural healing practices. In fact, treatments exist for nearly anything in the holistic world. The resources go far beyond the issue of Leaky Gut Syndrome. I have discovered that thousands of diseases deemed "incurable" by traditional medicine—diseases often muted by drugs that mask the symptoms—for which holistic medicine offers the hope of reversal. If you are suffering, I encourage you to explore what natural options may be available that your traditional doctor won't likely bring to your attention. It could be life-changing!

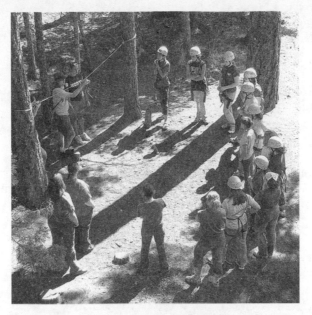

Me (far left) instructing high-ropes challenge course in 2004

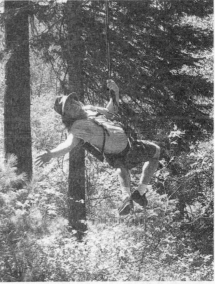

Riding low zipline 2004

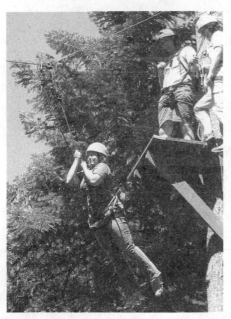

Operating zip line in 2004

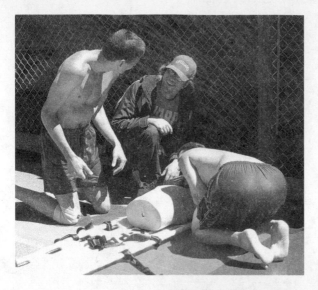

Teaching Red Cross lifeguard curriculum 2003

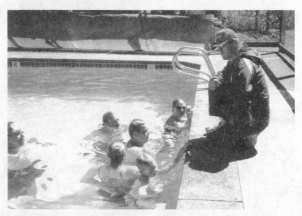

Red Cross lifeguard instructions 2003

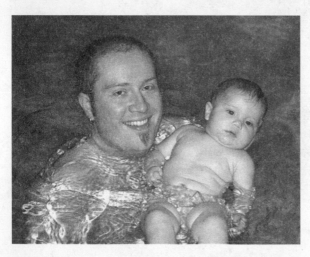

In 2009 at my heaviest (251 pounds), unaware sickness is growing

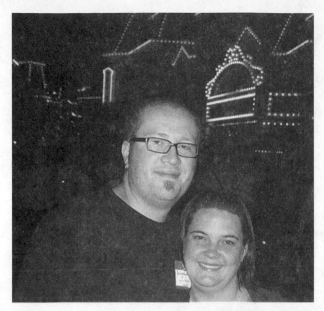

Vacationing at Disneyland in 2010, struggling with energy

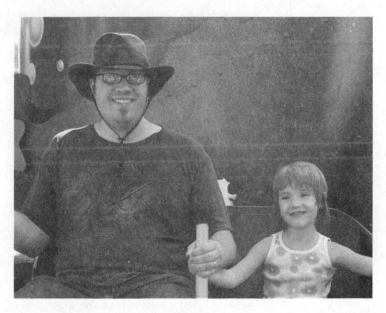

Disneyland 2010 with oldest daughter

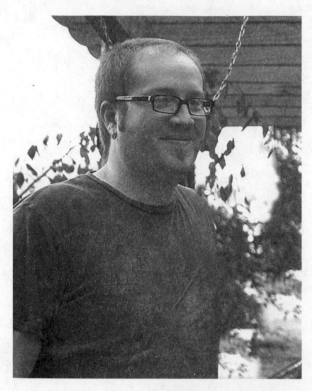

In 2011 I learn I have escalating fatty liver tissue

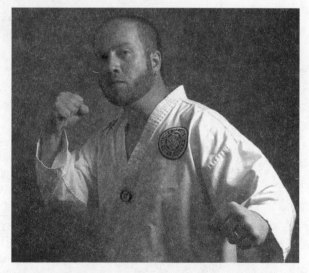

As a martial arts enthusiast, I lose fifty pounds in three months trying to reclaim health, while unknowingly burning adrenals

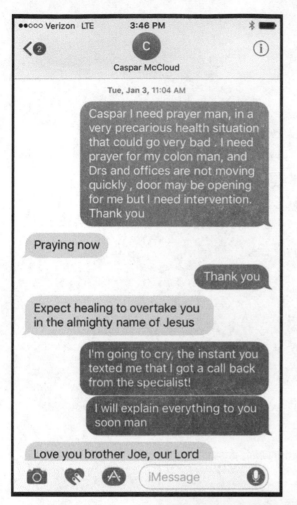

●●○○○ Verizon LTE   3:46 PM   ✶ ■

‹ 2   C   ⓘ
            Caspar McCloud

            Tue, Jan 3, 11:04 AM

Caspar I need prayer man, in a
very precarious health situation
that could go very bad . I need
prayer for my colon man, and
Drs and offices are not moving
quickly , door may be opening
for me but I need intervention.
Thank you

Praying now

                        Thank you

Expect healing to overtake you
in the almighty name of Jesus

I'm going to cry, the instant you
texted me that I got a call back
from the specialist!

I will explain everything to you
soon man

Love you brother Joe, our Lord

📷 💓 🅰 (iMessage) 🎤

Original screenshot from
Caspar McCloud's text
declaring I would be
healed [see chapter 1]

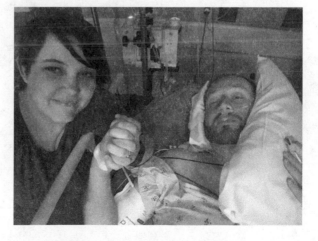

In hospital bed after
colon surgery, waking up
from anesthesia to see
my lovely wife Katherine

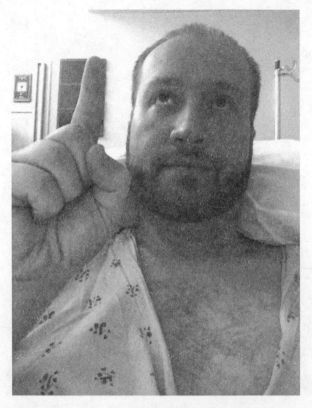

Somehow I knew the Lord would restore me

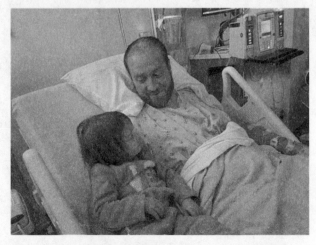

Visited by youngest daughter while at the hospital

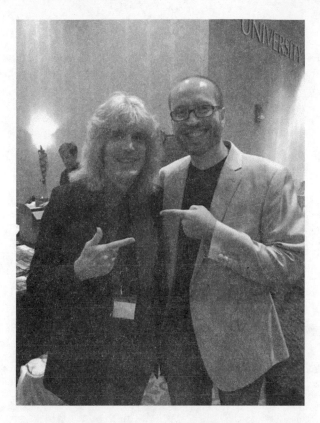

With Caspar. Regaining my health day by day, utilizing natural foods and supplements, following Dr. Joshua Vance's advice

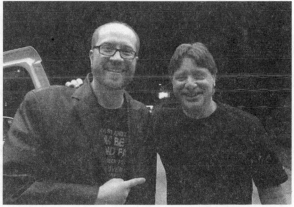

With my good friend (known to the public as 'the Fireman Prophet') Mark Taylor, who overcame similar health issues

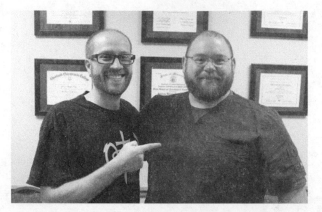

In Dr. Joshua Vance's office

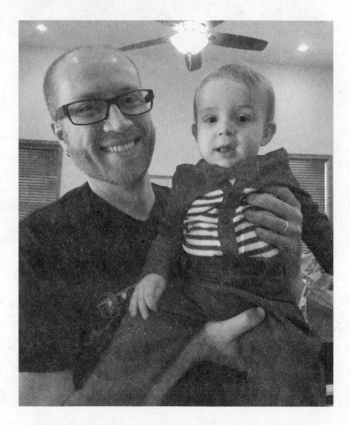

With fourth child and only son, at 180 pounds and feeling healthy for the first time in over a decade

FingerStick IgG 184 Food Panel

Joe Horn
D.O.B.:

REQUISITION:
COLLECTION DATE:
RUN DATE:

PINC

ALLETESS
MEDICAL LABORATORY

TEST	CLASS	TEST	CLASS	TEST	CLASS	TEST	CLASS
MEAT & POULTRY		**VEGETABLES**		**FRUITS**		**NUTS, SEEDS & OILS**	
Beef	0	Artichoke	0	Apple	1 *	Almond	0
Buffalo	0	Asparagus	0	Apricot	0	Brazil Nut	0
Chicken	0	Beets	0	Avocado	0	Canola	0
Duck	0	Bell Pepper	0	Banana	0	Cashew	0
Lamb	0	Broccoli	0	Blackberry	0	Chestnut	1 *
Pork	0	Brussel Sprouts	0	Blueberry	0	Chia Seed	0
Turkey	0	Cabbage	0	Cantaloupe	0	Cola	0
Venison	0	Carrot	0	Cherry	0	Flaxseed	1 *
		Cauliflower	0	Coconut	0	Hazelnut	0
FISH & SHELLFISH		Celery	0	Cranberry	0	Hemp	0
Anchovy	0	Cucumber	0	Date	0	Macadamia Nut	0
Bass	0	Eggplant	1 *	Fig	0	Pecan	0
Clam	0	Garlic	0	Grape	0	Pine Nut	0
Codfish	0	Green Bean	0	Grapefruit	0	Pistachio	0
Crab	0	Kale	0	Honeydew	0	Poppy Seed	1 *
Flounder	0	Kelp	0	Kiwi	1 *	Safflower	0
Haddock	0	Lettuce	0	Lemon	0	Sesame	1 *
Halibut	0	Mushroom	2 **	Lime	0	Sunflower Seed	0
Herring	0	Okra	0	Mango	0	Walnut	0
Lobster	0	Olive, Green	0	Orange	0		
Mackerel	0	Onion	0	Papaya	0	**HERBS, SPICES, FLAVORINGS**	
Mussel	0	Parsnip	0	Peach	0	Basil	0
Oyster	0	Potato	0	Pear	0	Bay Leaf	0
Perch	0	Potato, Sweet	0	Pineapple	1 *	Black Pepper	0
Red-Snapper	0	Pumpkin	0	Plum	0	Cilantro	0
Salmon	0	Radish	1 *	Raspberry	0	Cinnamon	1 *
Scallop	0	Spinach	0	Rhubarb	0	Cloves	0
Shrimp	0	Squash	0	Strawberry	0	Dill	0
Sole	0	Tomato	0	Tangerine	0	Fennel Seed	0
Squid	0	Turnip	0	Watermelon	0	Ginger	1 *
Swordfish	0	Zucchini	0			Ginseng	0
Trout	0			**BEVERAGES & MISC**		Horseradish	0
Tuna	0	**LEGUMES & PULSES**		Black Tea	0	Licorice	0
Walleye Pike	0	Black-eyed Peas	0	Carob	0	Mustard	0
		Chickpea	0	Cocoa	0	Nutmeg	1 *
GRAINS & STARCHES		Green Pea	0	Coffee	0	Oregano	1 *
Amaranth	0	Kidney Bean	0	Green Tea	0	Paprika	0
Arrowroot	0	Lentil	0	Honey	0	Parsley	0
Barley	1 *	Lima Bean	0	Yeast, Baker's	1 *	Peppermint	1 *
Bran	1 *	Navy Bean	0	Yeast, Brewer's	1 *	Rosemary	0
Buckwheat	0	Peanut	0			Sage	0
Corn	0	Soybean	0			Tarragon	1 *
Gluten	2 **					Thyme	0
Hops	0	**DAIRY & EGG**				Turmeric	0
Malt	0	Blue Cheese	2 **			Vanilla Bean	1 *
Millet	0	Casein	2 **				
Oats	0	Cheddar Cheese	1 *				
Quinoa	1 *	Cottage Cheese	2 **				
Rice	0	Egg, White	1 *				
Rye	0	Egg, Yolk	1 *				
Sorghum	0	Milk, Cow's	2 **				
Tapioca	0	Milk, Goat's	1 *				
Teff	1 *	Milk, Sheep's	2 **				
Wheat	2 **	Mozzarella Cheese	0				
		Swiss Cheese	0				
		Whey	2 **				
		Yogurt	3 ***				

Reference Range   G57 - 11658
0 = No Reactivity   1 = Low   2 = Moderate   3 = High

ALLETESS MEDICAL LABORATORY
74 Accord Park Drive, Norwell, MA 02061
800.225.5404 | +1.781.871.4426 | foodallergy.com
LABORATORY DIRECTOR:Gordon Siek, Ph.D. | C.L.I.A. # 22D0080258

Sample iGg panel showing my multiple food allergies

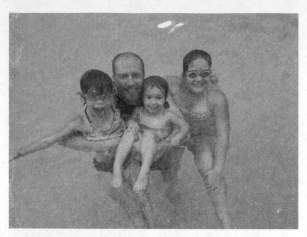

With the kids at the pool with energy to play

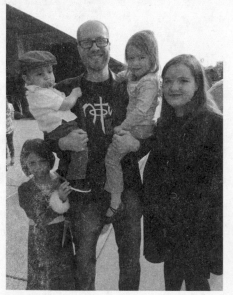

Attending a Christmas program with the kids in 2017

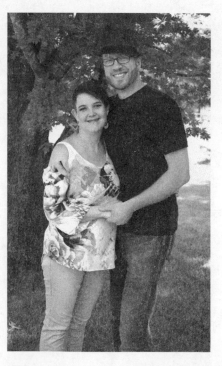

2017—with my beautiful wife Katherine, who carried me through the roughest times (who also lost thirty pounds since changing our eating habits)

10

Remember That First Ingredient

As mentioned previously, the first toxic ingredient in food is our attitude toward it. So naturally, the first step toward making a change for the better is to adjust our attitude toward our food. Up to this point, I have focused on showing you many of the ways our food system is in trouble. But, I can't bear to leave the issue there, with no message of hope. Likewise, I could not have bothered with this book if there wasn't something to share that would help you take control of your health and lifestyle. As part of this message of hope, it's necessary to revisit the concept of our attitude toward food. Once we've effectively adjusted this vital element, we can then apply practical applications that can be the beginning of a change.

The Importance of Nutritional Supplementation

By now, you're probably aware that most of the food for sale in a traditional grocery store is substandard in some way, either because of added toxic ingredients or diminished nutritional value prompted by mass food production. Changing your diet is a vital step in taking over your health, but just as important is dietary supplementation. As discussed in the previous chapter, when you have identified your deficiencies, it is important to make up the shortage with supplements. In addition, you should supplement your continued diet according to the advice of your holistic doctor, who will also be able to give you an idea of what kind you need based on your eating habits and physical condition.

In addition to knowing what types of supplements you should be taking, it is essential to choose a good-quality brand. Shopping for these can be confusing…and expensive. Some supplements, "even when taken in moderate daily doses, can be toxic."[146] Other brands do not have a good absorption rate. Sometimes, poor absorption is a result of the bonding agent of the capsule, and other times it is a result of the combination of supplements within the capsule. For a supplement to be well absorbed into the body, it not only has to be taken in a form the body can receive, but it has to be blended with elements that complement each other and allow the body to absorb the nutrition. This is one more area where working with your holistic doctor and locating (and continuing to watch the practices of) a trusted manufacturer will benefit you and ensure that the money you spend is maximized toward your good health.

Change Your Expectations

The lack of sugar, trans fats, excitotoxins, and other ingredients our bodies might be biologically addicted to can result, initially, in disappointment with whole foods in their nutritional simplicity. Recall that many of these ingredients cause signals to spark within the brain that creates almost a "high" associated with processed foods. This is a lot for a natural, wholesome, even organic food to compete with. This is where our challenge becomes our attitude. Anticipating an adjustment period and determining in advance to remain strong through this time of change will be the first great move you can make. Being ready for food to taste a little different, possibly even bland for a while, is your first defense. After your taste buds adapt, wholesome foods will become so dear to your heart that they will likely cause all processed treats to pale in comparison. This, for me, has been so true!

If you doubt what I'm saying, consider this: We consume, on average, volumes more sugar and salt then we used to, and our taste buds have likewise adapted. Recall when you were a child and put too much salt on your food. Do you remember how bitter it was—how it made your face pucker? Imagine what would happen if you were able to, using a time machine, "time-warp" somebody from a hundred years ago into our modern-day supermarket and feed him or her some of the snacks on our shelves. It's likely that the person would make the same face, as our current sodium levels are so much higher than they were a century years ago that the food would be way too "salty" to even consider palatable. Your taste buds have adapted over your lifetime, and this will reverse eventually with the correct habits and effort. But, especially at first, you must change your expectations and resolve to be content with food that may seem a little on the plain side. This is acceptable: It does not mean there is anything wrong with your food. It is possible that you're biologically addicted to the flavor enhancers and other ingredients you're used to experiencing in your food. But you are in control of this situation: you and *only* you. Remember, as previously stated, you must adopt the mind frame that food is not entertainment. It is simply fuel. If you begin to think in that old, familiar direction of wanting more excitement from your food, identify this deception for what it is: Do not allow this chemical trap to keep you from moving forward in a healthy direction! If you want entertainment, make up your mind to find it another way. Your food is only meant to fuel your body. The biggest change you will have to make is being willing to accept a blander blend of meal time and snack time selections until you learn how to replace the flavor with things that are not harmful and your taste buds adapt to a newer, healthier diet. Once they have, processed foods will eventually taste terrible.

Additionally, as you begin to cook healthier food, beyond the adaptation of your taste buds, you will soon learn how to season your foods using healthy ingredients in ways that bring back a delicious and guilt-free flavor. Your food will require more effort as you begin to make more meals from scratch, but the biggest issue with this type of cooking, contrary to many people's beliefs, is not that it is too hard or even that it takes very much time. It is that *we haven't learned how, so we are intimidated by the idea of doing it.* But almost no healthy food is cheap, easy, and fast. A person must choose which of those attributes is a priority and follow accordingly. You will likely find that cooking from scratch is easier when you take a little bit of time to plan. As you develop new, tried-and-true recipes, it becomes easier over time. Additionally, many staple ingredients are significantly less expensive than boxed meal kits, etc., so you may find over time that you are *saving money.* The secret is to hang in there and keep trying until you find some easy home-made recipes your family enjoys.

Dr. Mercola states:

Someone has to spend quality time in the kitchen to prepare high-quality meals for your health. If you rely on processed inexpensive foods you will simply exchange convenience and short-term cash savings for long-term health miseries. Swapping your processed food diet for one that focuses on real, whole foods may seem like a radical idea, but it's a necessity if you value your health.[147]

A Worthy Cause

As I previously stated, it's important that you take away from this book a message of hope. You *can* change what you are doing, a little step at a time. You can switch off the timebomb in your gut! Many resources are available to help you with this transition. Remember, we live in the age of knowledge. We simply have to put some effort into finding these resources and utilizing them. But when it comes time to invest in the change, many worry that they won't find the time for follow-through.

For a moment, think about how you spend your time. The average American spends ten hours per day plugged into some kind of media, five of which are spent in front of the television. In addition to this, we spend, on average, roughly an hour on the Internet, nearly three hours listening to the radio, and over an hour on our phones.[148] Perhaps you don't fall into these categories, but many Americans do. Reflecting over the issues presented in this book, surely there must be *something* you can cut from your busy schedule to make time to prioritize food preparation for yourself and your family. I encourage you to talk with your family, possibly even share with them some of the things you've read. If they understand why their menu is changing, they may be even supportive enough to help (depending on the circumstances, age of family members, etc.). The meals you present to them at first may not be what they're used to, especially if you're one of the folks who will now be trying to learn to cook, but many studies show that people report the same food as tasting better when they perceive it to be prepared with love.[149] This means that your effort to fix a home-cooked, healthy meal prepared with their best interests in mind can actually be a hit at the dinner table, despite your possible lack of skill. Again, until my health *required* me to prepare my own meals, I was always the guy who said, "Nah, I don't know what I'm doing in the kitchen."

Considering the health risks involved with eating substandard food, many people respond that they will "find the time" to make a change for their own future and the future of their children. It is a journey well worth it.

Starting a New Journey

Just as is the case with many changes we decide to make, getting the ball rolling is the hardest. The most effective way to begin this change is with a safe detox from processed foods. Talk to your holistic doctor about what kind of detox will be best for you. We will discuss in upcoming pages some tips that may help as you go about this process, but this is not to take the place of your holistic doctor's advice, as individual needs can vary. In addition, some recommended steps for change are listed in the next chapter—you might start to adopt these while following the detox process. Take these steps as few as one or two at a time if necessary. Remember to give yourself a break—drastic change does not happen overnight, and it's likely that the food habits you are currently practicing have taken a lifetime to build. Remember that a couple of good, manageable, affordable, and sustainable steps in the right direction will make a better change for you in the long term than a radical, expensive crash course in dietary change that becomes too much to manage and therefore is not followed through. Begin with a small number of these recommended steps, and as you grow comfortable, proceed at your own pace. Overall, long-term success is what matters, so give yourself grace.

At the start of such a lifestyle change, many people might be tempted to make sudden, radical overhauls to their diet, which can be great. The issue with this, however, can be that many people launch changes that, over time, they cannot keep. If this weren't true, we would all be more successful in keeping our New Year's resolutions than we are. When the "new" wears off, the busy mom may find herself tempted to return to old routines, succumbing to the fear that it's too much to keep up with.

Likewise, the entrepreneurial man, juggling payroll, employees, and too many work projects may give in and return to his old habits of driving through the fast-food window at a chain restaurant for a cheeseburger at lunch time, wishing he could have changed his life, but resigned to the idea that he will never find the time to do so. Taking these steps in smaller increments ensures that you acclimate to one or two changes, and when they have become a lifestyle, you're ready to take on a couple more changes. In this way, you really *can* make a change and keep it.

Here are some simple rules that you can begin following immediately that will help you as you begin to eliminate dangerous food. They may seem oversimplified to some, but they are geared toward empowering the average person in simple ways to make healthy changes, even if you're not yet finished reading this book. There are many other things you will probably eventually decide to change about your diet, but this will get you started:

1. Begin to plan your meals. The meal plan doesn't have to be overwhelming. Start by keeping it simple. Choose two new recipes to try that do not list processed foods as ingredients, and try them. Make double batches, so that you don't have to cook at each meal if you're not used to cooking. When you feel that you have been successful at these two recipes, choose another two to try. Make it a process you repeat until you have a collection of recipes you feel good about.

2. Once you have established a plan of nutrition with your holistic doctor, follow that plan as though your health depends on it (because it does!). Avoid things you know will make you sick.

3. Stay hydrated! In order to calculate how much water you need, "Take your weight in pounds. Divide the weight in half. The result is the number of ounces of water you should drink daily."[1]

4. To stay hydrated, be watchful of what you're drinking. Many sports drinks that market their ability to "hydrate" are big culprits for sneaking sugar into your daily diet.

5. Take the supplements that you and your holistic doctor agree upon.

6. Get plenty of sleep.

7. Eat at regular intervals; don't over eat or allow yourself to "starve" for long periods of time.

8. Shop the perimeter of the grocery store. This simple rule will not ensure that you are buying only organic food, but it will immediately get you out of the junk/processed-food zone. Think about this: You typically enter the store in the produce section. Of course, there are concerns with some produce as we discussed early in the book, but, as the USDA report stated, the worst produce is still better than most of the products that are available throughout the rest of the store. You can become more particular about produce later, when you're ready to take that on. For now, enter in the produce area. Then, walking the perimeter should take you through the meat department, the dairy, and the bread area. Although these departments aren't guaranteed to have faultless products, it is a sure thing that the only "whole foods" to be found in the supermarket will be located in these sections. Avoid the middle of the store. This is where the cereals, chips, cookies, pre-boxed dinners, and all the very worst foods are located. Again, buy your food from the perimeter.

9. In addition, buy fresh produce whenever possible, and try to eliminate choosing anything in cans. Select frozen produce over canned any time fresh is not available (the chemicals used to prepare the cans for food are not listed on the nutrition label, but are also harmful, whereas frozen products usually

undergo a smaller amount of chemical exposure). For things like kidney beans, black beans, or pinto beans, buy them raw and rinse them before use, likewise avoiding the canned products. Or preferably, buy them dry (or in bulk) and boil them.

10. Wash all produce. Many concerns with produce have to do with the chemicals sprayed on them during the growth and harvest process. Wash them thoroughly!

11. When possible, remove peel from produce. The peel serves as an additional shielding layer over your food, protecting it from dangerous chemicals. As you learn more about which fruits and vegetables in your area are available organically at an affordable price, you can adjust your buying habits as you see fit.

12. Buy local whenever available. Anytime you can, buy from a local source so that you can be more informed about the process under which your food was produced.

13. Don't shop while you are hungry. Not only will this keep to a minimum the temptation to buy junk food or processed food, it will also save on your budget!

14. Don't shop while you are emotional. Remember, the worst foods are marketed toward your need to feel comfort, happy, or indulged. *Don't fall for it.* Shop with the calculated understanding that food is *fuel.*

15. If you are trying to lose weight, resist the temptation to skip meals.

16. When you can, exercise. Even if it means getting out from behind your desk on your lunch break and taking a brisk walk through the neighborhood, the physical activity and mental break will do your health a world of good. Exercise isn't covered in this book, but that doesn't mean I don't believe physical activity is a vital part of overall health.

17. If you must decide between two types of processed foods, choose the one with the least toxic ingredients and eat a smaller amount (for example, instead of eating an entire lunch in the setting, just eat a snack-sized amount), putting off a full meal until you can get to a place where you will have access to more nutritious food.

18. Learn to appreciate the simplicity of nutritious food. Give your palate time to adapt to whole foods. See clean, healthy food and appreciate it as a high-quality, nutrient-rich product instead of seeking high-sugar or high-fat foods that stimulate the taste buds.

19. If you can, start a garden. True, this is easier said than done. However, kids enjoy having a garden, and there are many great resources for growing healthy foods—even in small spaces or urban settings. The Internet is a great resource as well. This doesn't have to mean that you are trying to grow your *entire food source* on the back porch of a two-bedroom apartment in the middle of the city. It is only a suggestion that you might give it a try, with the possibility of producing *some* of your own food. You and your kids may really enjoy it.

20. As you become more comfortable with these changes, take up label reading as a new habit. Watch for healthy ingredients and weed toxic ingredients out of your diet one or two at a time. When you've completely cut one ingredient from your diet, choose a new one.

21. Don't mistake "organic" food for "healthy" food. For example, you can go to a health store and buy a box of "organic" cookies. But they are still made with flour, sugar, chocolate, and other ingredients that aren't good for you. Cookies are not a health food, whether they're "organic" or otherwise. An "organic" box of cookies would likely run you five or six

dollars, where a box of Oreos might cost three. This is part of the reason many people adopt the misconception that they can't afford to eat organically. But, as I've said throughout this book, we must adjust our thinking. We are *overhauling* our lifestyle, not *trading out* one dangerous, expensive snack for another. Just as I had to let go of the idea that I would go *backward* to health (as I mentioned at the beginning of the book), the answer is letting go of the cookies altogether.

22. Avoid the following ingredients we've already discussed. Because these toxic ingredients are often being relisted (and hidden!) under new or different names, it is wise to occasionally search for new aliases to the following list of ingredients, to ensure avoidance.

- High-fructose corn syrup (HFCS)
- Synthetic trans fats
- Monosodium glutamate (MSG)
- Artificial colors
- Artificial sweeteners
- Sodium nitrate and Sodium nitrate
- Artificial flavors
- Butylated hydroxyanisole (BHA), butylated hydrozytoluene (BHT), and tertiary butylhydroquinone (TBHQ)
- Sodium benzoate and benzoic acid
- Potassium bromate
- Sulfites
- Other preservatives
- Other excitotoxins as you learn to identify them
- Meats containing antibiotics or hormones (nearly everything at the standard grocery store)
- Dairy products containing antibiotics or hormones

Detoxing Safely

It is important to remember to detox safely. Just as I did when I went through withdrawal sickness after visiting that first holistic doctor, it is possible to overload your liver and kidneys during the detox process. The process should be done safely, *not necessarily quickly*. Talk to your naturopath about the safest and most efficient plan for getting your body through a healthy detox, and follow it to the letter.

Grocery Overhaul

At this point, you might be ready to throw away all your old food and rush to the grocery store to replace it with healthy alternatives. Before you do that, however, it is important that you don't accidentally replace that food with *other* unhealthy food. Deciding to transition slowly, learning as you go, replacing a few healthy ingredients and adopting a few new, homemade recipes at a time, will help you create a more sustainable, long-term lifestyle that will also help you ease your budget into the new changes.

As stated many times in this book, the only way to fully guarantee that you are receiving the healthiest and purest food possible is by finding local, organic producers whom you trust—and then stick to using only their products. That said, many people who live in urban communities may not have access to such local producers. For these people, I am including some tips on how to make the best grocery store selections possible.

Produce: When choosing produce, if you are unable to buy organic, select dark, rich colors, as this often indicates nutritional content, and choose produce of all colors, since varying colors indicate varying nutrients.[151] When possible, avoid bruised or damaged fruits and vegetables, and always wash them. If fresh produce is not available and a certain fruit or vegetable is a must-have ingredient, frozen is a better option than canned. As stated previously, even if the ingredients on a can seem simple, the companies do not list the chemicals used to prepare the can itself for food content.

Dairy Products: Most grocery stores now carry an organic option for most dairy products. Try to purchase from the closest dairies and investigate their practices as thoroughly as possible. Choose rGBH and other hormone-free products whenever available, or even substitute ingredients if an adequate product can't be found, such as trading one variety of cheese for another. Whenever possible, it is important that animals involved are fed their native diets.[152]

Meats: As with dairy products, it is important to choose products free of hormones, antibiotics, and other drugs. Choose products from food animals who were fed their native diets.[153] Determining whether a meat contains gratuitous hormones, antibiotics, or other drugs may be difficult, especially if you're purchasing from a grocery store. It doesn't hurt to ask store management if they know the product's origin. (Example: One local supermarket near me, at first glance, appears to have commercially imported, low-quality meat, but to my surprise, after talking with management, I learned that it purchases grass-fed beef from a farm located just seventy miles away.)

As with all products you purchase at the grocery store, watch out for common, deceptive manufacturer's label tricks, which will be highlighted in the next chapter.

11

The Label Game

Though labels are a great tool, they're not your safety net. As always, you must be your own vigilant guardian. What we need to ask beyond the question "is this *label* trustworthy?" should be "is this *manufacturer* trustworthy?" As discussed repeatedly throughout this book, many manufacturers have tried, still try, and will continue to try to sneak harmful ingredients into their products under newer, more ambiguous names. Understanding how to read the labels and what to watch for is an important part of this, but building a trusted repertoire of tried-and-true brands is equally as important in understanding labels.

Beyond this, remember that depending on a label is still part of the problem outlined in this book. Relying on labels is indirectly *still* expecting someone else to do our product policing for us. And, as previously discussed, this is not a reliable solution. What we need, in an ideal world, are supermarkets filled with foods that need no labels. Hoping that "they" have labeled their products with integrity is still feeding the larger idea that "they" are going to be honest with you or take care of you.

In 2008, Michael Pollan wrote an article encouraging consumers to limit their purchases to food products that include no more than five ingredients and no ingredients with names that can't be pronounced.

The shortened, brilliant mantra resulting from his statement became: "If you can't pronounce it, don't eat it."[154]

Dr. Mark Hyman put it this way in a recent article: "Eat from the right plant—if it was made in a plant stay away, if it was grown on a plant it is probably okay."[155]

Or perhaps it is better said by Dr. Mercola, "While many well-meaning nutritionists will teach you the importance of reading food labels, the easiest way to eat healthy is to stick with foods that need no food label at all.… When was the last time you saw an ingredients list on a grass-fed steak or a bunch of broccoli?"[156]

While this is great advice, sometimes it is easier said than done. (And, as we have covered in this book, even many simple foods are not without their issues.) On the other hand, it is unavoidable at certain times to purchase products that come packaged with a label. For those instances, understanding nutrition labels and the phrases commonly used on them will help you understand what you're really buying when you are purchasing food and beverages.

Many, however, dread the part of this journey that requires learning to efficiently read and understand the nutrition labels on our food. While reading the nutrition label is a vital part of choosing safe food, it is equally important to understand what we are watching *for*. But how do we do this effectively when it seems that food companies are constantly changing their labeling? The challenge can be overwhelming for the shopper. For example: A person might finally think that he or she has eliminated sugar from his or her diet, only to find that "trusted" brands ("tried and trues") included a disguised, more harmful version of sugar all along (remember, if it ends in "-ose" it's a sugar)? How do we get ahead of this?

The first step is to understand the labeling. Are labels friend or foe? They can be both, and unfortunately, it falls on us, the consumers, as our own vigilant guards, to determine which we are dealing with on a case-by-case basis. As buying trends change, many food companies change their products to meet demands. Unfortunately, many manufacturers also adjust their labeling to *appear as though* they have adjusted the food product inside, when it is the same product previously marketed under a different label. I remember seeing this firsthand when one of the latest dietary trends began to take off. I remember seeing "Gluten-Free!" on all kinds of products throughout the supermarket. Shelves were filled with packages bearing this label all around me. Products such as eggs that have no way of containing gluten were even being proudly advertised as having no gluten. Since gluten is a derivative of wheat, it wouldn't be found in eggs anyway! But I assure you that as consumer demands change, at the very least, so does the labeling. Gluten-free eggs and low-carb or carb-free chicken are only a few examples of these labeling tricks. Similarly, as awareness about certain ingredients escalates, food conglomerates adjust their labeling accordingly, hiding certain ingredients in plain sight and creating new "trend phrases" that lend credibility to the same old products that many have already deemed unwise to consume. This doesn't necessarily mean the product inside is any different than before the label changed. Learning to analyze the information on a nutrition label and separating the "tricks" from the truth is one of the hardest but most rewarding steps in this process.

More often than we care to admit, labels we read and want to trust are merely another pathway on which our emotional assumption of comfort and peace can allow us to support a market based on big business. Often, we know the answer about a product before we pick it up off the shelf to look at the label. In situations like this, go with your gut.

Reading the front label on a product will not give you all the information you need. Unfortunately, claims on the front of a product sometimes contradict the *actual* information on the back of it (a practice that, in my opinion, should be illegal), where the nutrition and ingredient information are listed. For example, in my early days of trying to overhaul my family's diet, I naively purchased a bag of frozen tilapia. The front cover displayed a picture of a fisherman in a boat out on the water, and at the bottom corner of the package were the words: "Packaged in America." But later, when I read the back of the container, I learned that the fish were a "product of China" and had been imported, then subsequently repackaged for retail sale in America. The label held no further details as to the origin of the product. These labeling cons are just a few of many ways that consumers have to watch their backs.

Here are some common label-reading mistakes that steer people wrong when they are beginning a lifestyle overhaul.

1. Understand the allotted serving size on a nutrition label. Never assume that the nutrition label is giving you the information for the *entire container*. For example, a bottle of fruit juice may have a nutrition label that gives information about its contents, but at the top of the label there will be a number to indicate how many serving sizes are *included in that bottle*. If that number is two, then by drinking the *entire* jar of fruit juice, you are *consuming* two servings. In this particular case, this means that anything else listed on that label has to be doubled in order to accurately determine the number of nutrients, sugar, or other elements within that juice.

2. Remember that percentages of daily values (DV) on nutrition labels are based on a 2,000-calorie-per-day diet for healthy adults. For children, pregnant or breastfeeding women, individuals with sedentary lifestyles, or people with special medical or dietary needs, this number is not necessarily accurate.

3. Understand that the goal of the listed daily value (DV) is a different indicator for you depending on what the ingredient is listed next to. For example, if it is labeling saturated fat, which is an ingredient to avoid, you will want this number, as you add up all consumed foods throughout your entire day to stay as close to "0" as possible, because it is not a healthy ingredient. However,

for a healthy ingredient, such as vitamin C, throughout the day you would want the total number to eventually equal 100.

4. Watch for ingredients that hide in plain sight. "When the Nutrition Facts label says of food contains '0 g' of *trans* fat, but includes 'partially hydrogenated oil' in the ingredient list, it means that food contains trans fat, but less than 0.5 g of trans fat per serving."[157] As mentioned previously, another example of such a situation is when several types of sugars are used to keep any one form of sugar from escalating to the top of the ingredients list. It is important to know all the varying names of toxic ingredients.

5. Because of the variation between ingredients, manufacturing processes, and even individuals consuming products (our bodies all digest food differently because of that unique gut flora we discussed), calorie counts on nutrition labels are estimates at best. Jeanine Barone of *Berkeley Wellness* with the University of California said in a 2016 article:

The FDA allows food companies wide latitude in the accuracy of the calories listed on package labels—20 percent in either direction. That means if the label says 200 calories per serving, it could be 240 calories or 160 calories or anything in between. What's more, the FDA doesn't do any systematic policing of labels to ensure that calorie counts meet even that lax degree of accuracy. The responsibility for label accuracy remains with the food companies, from national manufacturers to regional or local vendors. It basically works on the honor system.[158]

Barone's article goes on to explain that in a perfect world, finished products would be tested individually in a lab to determine accurate calorie counts for each food product, but unfortunately, most companies simply combine caloric contributions from each of the ingredients and then give a final caloric estimate that is printed on the label. If manufacturers are receiving accurate information about their ingredients, this *could* be reliable. Again, this relies on individual consumer judgment based on the trustworthiness of the brand. If we are not counting calories or attempting to lose weight, this may seem like less of a concern, but for those with diabetes or other illness, this discrepancy could pose a health risk. Additionally, if this is how the calorie counts are being policed (or not), then who is to say that this principle doesn't potentially apply to nearly any other information on the label? If anything is critical to your health that you're watching labels for, make sure you are buying from trusted brands. This problem can be even worse at restaurants, where chefs may vary serving sizes slightly.[159]

6. Anytime you notice a new ingredient, investigate it. It could be a dangerous one that you've already weeded out of your diet that is attempting to reemerge under a new name.

What Label Phrases Really Mean

Trying to improve diet and remove toxic chemicals can be tricky, especially at first, with so many labeling terms plastered across every product in the grocery store. Once a person has decided to improve the food quality in his or her household, it can be difficult to separate a good food decision from a waste of money. To help demystify some these difficulties, here is a list of claims often made on food products and what they really mean.

1. "USDA Inspected"—When a label states a product is "USDA Inspected," it means the quality and size have passed standards

regulated by the United States Department of Agriculture. This label, however, does not address manufacturing methods, so much can still be ambiguous about the product's origin, especially in products that have been imported.

2. "Free" labels, such as "Gluten-Free" or "Cholesterol-Free"—If a product claims that it is "*anything*-free," then it should be exactly that. However, with any kind of label that advertises the product inside to be fully "free" of something, investigate the product before you spend the extra money for the product. (Recall the "gluten-free" eggs.) Take, for example, Dr. Steven Devries' comment about "No Cholesterol Peanut Butter," to which his response was, "the food never contained cholesterol in the first place, i.e. 'no cholesterol peanut butter.' Cholesterol is only found in animal products. Plant derived food never has cholesterol…. Don't pay extra for plant products with this label."[160]

3. Whole-grain labels—Watch for labels with words and phrases like "Multi-Grain" or "Made with Whole Grains." Unless the manufacturer puts a percentage of whole grains used on the label, this could be a scam. Made "with" could mean that sometime during the manufacturing process, an unspecified amount of whole grains was added to a recipe also filled with regular white flour. If you're looking for a product made completely of whole grains, watch for a label that says "100% Whole Grains."

4. "No Sugar Added"—This label can be counterproductive in that it means no extra sugar has been added to the product. This does not mean that the product contains *no sugar*. It essentially places the consumers back at square one, forcing them to decipher whether they are holding a product that *would* contain sugar. For example, this is a popular label on applesauce. But because apples are the key ingredient in applesauce, obviously there is some natural sugar in the product.

5. "Grass-Fed"—To label a food animal as simply "Grass-Fed" does not mean that no drugs or hormones were used on the animal. It only means that the animal's primary food source, after weaning, was grass or foraging, not grains.[161] If you are looking for beef that is completely grass-fed, look for the label "100% Grass-Fed." However, "Pasture-Raised" or "Pastured" means that the animal "spent at least some time outdoors on pasture,"[162] with no regulatory minimum imposed.

6. "Antibiotic-Free"—This label means that the manufacturer claims the food animal "received no antibiotics over its lifetime."[163] To be certified as USDA organic, food animals have to meet this standard.

7. "Hormone-Free," "Raised without Hormones," and "No Hormones Administered"—Because federal law prohibits hormones to be used within food hogs or food poultry, this label is meaningless and unnecessary, similar to the earlier-mentioned "gluten-free eggs." However, hormones are still permitted in the use of beef and dairy cattle.[164] It is important to note that these labels indicate it is the manufacturer's claim that no hormones were ever used on the involved food animal.

8. "Organic"—This word appearing by itself, without the phrase "USDA Certified" beside it, can be misleading, because unless the USDA has qualified standards for a specific product, the word "Organic" is exactly that: merely a word on the label. An example of this is found on seafood. The US government has not completed a standard for certifying seafood as "Organic."[165] Thus, any seafood advertised as such is possibly doing so independently of the USDA as a marketing scheme. On the other hand, many manufacturers who want to label their products as "Organic" have quantified their own standards and submitted them to the USDA for approval. Because of this, the word "Organic" on a label doesn't necessarily have to be a cause

for distrust, as it could mean a manufacturer is trying to create a higher level of standard. But, if you're looking for a grade of organic that meets with *preset governmental standards*, it must include "USDA" on the label.[166]

This all being said, the "USDA 100% Organic" label means the manufacturers claim (and the USDA certifies) that every ingredient used in producing the enclosed product is organic. "USDA Organic" indicates that 95 percent of the ingredients used to make the final product are organic. "Made with Organic Ingredients" specifies the product was made "with a minimum of 70% organic ingredients with strict restrictions on the remaining 30%, including no GMOs."[167]

9. "Organic" labels on animal products—For milk to be "Certified Organic," the dairy cow must be fed at least 30 percent of its food at pasture for at least 120 days, and must receive no antibiotics or hormones, with the supplementary feed being organic and free from animal byproducts. The "Organic" label on poultry means that only organic feed is allowed, and that no medication or vaccination may be used. This causes increased casualties, which contributes to the higher cost of organic poultry.[168]

10. "Cage-Free"—This designation, concerning poultry, can mean very little. All it really indicates is that the birds did not live in a cage. However, many of the big, commercial poultry farms raise their birds in large chicken houses that contain no *actual cages*.

11. "Free-Range"—The USDA, as of now, has only regulated this phrase for the use of poultry. These words on any other product are a simple claim of the manufacturer, with no USDA regulations to back it. It simply means that the food animal had access to the outdoors for an unspecified amount of time each day.[169]

12. "Natural"—This label goes on products that do not contain artificial ingredients or preservatives, and the ingredients are only minimally processed. Items in this category may, however, contain

antibiotics, growth hormones, or similar chemicals.[170] Foods bearing the label "All Natural" or "100% Natural" are regulated the same way as those labeled "Natural."[171] Many people see the word "Natural" on a label and mistake it for "Organic," but this is a mistake, and can result in spending money on products that have a lower standard than what you want.

13. "Certified Humane"—When featured on poultry packaging, this label lets consumers know that the manufacturer has met standards set by the Humane Society for the humane treatment of birds. For example, these standards say the birds can be kept indoors at all times, but must be able to perform many of their "natural behaviors such as nesting, perching, and dust bathing. There are requirements for stocking density and number of perches and nesting boxes. Forced molting through starvation is prohibited, but beak cutting is allowed."[172]

14. "Animal Welfare Approved"—This label on poultry means that "beak cutting is prohibited, birds must molt naturally, they are cage free and have continuous access to outdoor perching. Stocking density, space and nesting boxes are regulated as well."[173]

15. "Fresh"—With very little regulation applied to this word, this is most often an arbitrary claim made by the manufacturer. The only standard the USDA has applied to the word "fresh" is as it pertains to whether poultry has been frozen.[174]

Organic Products

Not only is the USDA "Certified Organic" label, at this time, the "most meaningful label on your food, in terms of upholding specific government requirements,"[175] it guarantees that crops are grown without synthetic fertilizers, synthetic pesticides, or sewage sludge and are not genetically engineered or eradicated. Further, it ensures that food animals are given organic feed containing no animal byproducts, synthetic hormones, or antibiotics; are raised in a setting conducive to nature; and are not cloned.[176]

Beyond this, the Sanderson case discussed earlier and others like it prove that organic farmers are uniting to preserve the "Organic" label and its integrity. This means that whereas one might doubt the policing of USDA-regulated labels, at this time, many manufacturers *behind* these labels are holding each other accountable. The Sanderson instance, wherein poultry was treated with illegal substances, was discovered by organic farmers, who promptly filed suit. Does this mean the "Organic" label is the new answer to all our dietary problems? Not necessarily. It simply indicates that it represents a group of people who are trying to bring about a revolution in the quality of our food.

This is where the consumers now hold some power. If we can support the organic movement and keep the product integrity that it represents intact, it could be the beginning of a real change for our entire food marketing and manufacturing industry—a change we really need. While it may seem that individually boycotting products sold by the large manufacturers will never make a difference, this is proving untrue. If our meager, isolated dollars spent or withheld here and there were not enough to speak for themselves, we wouldn't see large conglomerates like Nestlé buying up companies like Atrium Innovations, the makers of Garden of Life Supplements. Companies like Coca-Cola wouldn't bother with subordinate companies like Honest Tea and Odwalla; Kellogg wouldn't own Bear Naked and Kashi; and the M&M and Mars Corporation would not bother owning Seeds of Change. The fact that these powerhouse companies are dividing their resources to introduce, invest in, and manufacture healthier foods strongly suggests they see where our money is going and will fight to gain those sales. Make no mistake: These companies are after your money. As vigilant consumers, we must fight to keep sales honest and products reputable. Right now, some of our strongest advocates are organic farmers and local sellers.

While we may feel like our dollars are small compared to the millions these large corporations see daily, our spending habits apparently are strong enough to turn the heads of the powers that be within these businesses. Even more, it is enough to make a *huge* difference for local, organic farmers.

The general movement toward organic food is being displayed in many ways. For example, a significant number of young professionals with college degrees are trading their professional jobs for a future in farming. "Sixty-nine percent of…surveyed young farmers had college degrees—significantly higher than the general population."[177] Further, "a survey conducted by the National Young Farmers Coalition…shows that the majority of young farmers did not grow up in agricultural families."[178]

I find this information encouraging. There is a movement stirring in the air right now, a sweeping change within our food industry. A new, radical type of farmer is on the rise, holding organic standards high and keeping comrades accountable. He is educated, young, passionate, and resourceful.

His female counterpart is just as dedicated. She can be found in the wee hours of the morning harvesting greens before the sun can rise to wilt her crop. She makes sacrifices for the movement she believes in. "Finances can be tight. The women admit they've given up higher standards of living to farm."[179]

These up-and-coming farmers are a key ingredient in a movement that must happen for our society's health to change. They are marketing to small local grocery stores and restaurants, and they're selling their harvest at farmers' markets. The economy is responding on several levels: Restaurants are purchasing locally again; grocers are introducing local food-buying programs; and consumers are buying locally and asking for locally sourced products in the places they shop. These indicators are proof that we are on the cusp of change. Yet, these changes could be thwarted before they are fully brought about if we don't make certain that our voices are heard.

Tips for Organic and Scratch Cooking

Let's now narrow our focus from the wide-ranging issues concerning healthier, safer food production and the healthy ways to select our groceries to a much more specific topic, one that can be summed up with one question: Once we've stocked our cabinets and refrigerators with natural and healthy foods, what's next? Ours is the generation of fast food and quick fixes, Happy Meals and Stovetop Stuffing. How do we begin to make the transition from "drive through" or "just add water" to measuring, mixing, and preparing to come up with meals our families will not just eat, but enjoy?

The biggest obstacle for many who are asking these questions is where and how to start. Once we get used to the new routine and have formed new habits, creativity flows more easily. The biggest change most of us struggle with is making the effort to plan. If you can try (I know this is much easier said than done!) to think even a day ahead, you may find it gets easier. Another bonus to this new way of life is the money saved by packing your family's lunches rather than spending money on convenience foods.

Here are some tips that might help you tackle this new challenge:

- **Make enough for extra meals.** When you make dinner, fix enough so that there are leftovers you can pack in your family's lunches for the following day as well. This may cause extra dirty dishes to come home in lunch bags, but the money you save and knowing your family isn't eating fast food at lunch time will be well worth the adjustment.
- **Invest in a slow cooker.** Any meals you previously would have made with canned beans, such as chili or burritos, can now be planned the night before. Rinse the beans and soak them overnight in the fridge. The next morning while you're making your coffee or tea, rinse the beans again, place them in the slow cooker, and

set it to cook on the temperature setting recommended by your chosen recipe. When you arrive home, the beans will be ready to serve—without all the chemicals of canned beans.

- **Invest in a bread maker.** Homemade bread requires very few ingredients—and if you buy organic ingredients, you can eat bread guilt free (as long as you don't have a sensitivity to wheat or some other reason to cause you to need to avoid eating bread. If you are allergic to wheat, ask your holistic doctor what type of flour would be best for you, as there many non-wheat flours are available. I personally like rice flour.) Keep the ingredients near the bread machine so that in the morning, you can get the bread started while you're waiting for your coffee or tea to brew. You will come home to a house that smells like freshly baked bread, and it's bread you can feel good about eating.

- **Rethink your cereal.** Replace the high-sugar cereals with organic granola or other grain cereal that your gut does not adversely react to for a quick breakfast. Ask your holistic doctor for recommendations based on your dietary needs.

- **Eat eggs for protein.** Once or twice a week, hard boil eggs for a quick, on-the-go protein snack. Write the date you boiled them on the shells to keep up with which eggs were boiled on what day.

- **Invest in a high-quality, electric pressure cooker.** My wife and I have found that we can cook meals that normally would have taken all day in about an hour. Some of our favorites include bone-broth stew (great for healing the gut), hard pinto or kidney beans, and roast beef. The wonderful thing about this is when she hasn't had time to plan ahead and place a meal in the crockpot, she still can create a home-made meal for our family at the last minute. We prefer the electric-style pressure cooker, because it regulates its own pressure and doesn't pose the burn risks of an old-fashioned, stove-top-style pressure cooker.

- **Befriend your butcher.** Many people who raise their own meat don't want the bones, and some butchers will save them if they know they have a buyer. Consider negotiating an inexpensive purchase of the bones of locally raised, organically fed food animals tomake bone broth. I actually get mine free from a local butcher who would otherwise toss them in the garbage—and they make incredible bone broth!

- **Join an online food or recipe club.** Many people get online to exchange recipes and tips for bringing healthy food to their families' tables. In fact, it's a good idea to utilize the Internet often for all sorts of help with organizing, planning, and creating healthy meals.

- **Invest in a water filter.** This will keep you and your family from ingesting chemicals introduced into the water supply if your home is not on a well system.

- **Use your freezer and consider buying an additional one.** When you know you'll be heading into a busy time, prepare foods ahead and freeze them. In fact, it's a great idea to keep two or three backup dinners frozen at all times. That will curb your desire to eat out when you're having a busy week or otherwise haven't had the time to plan ahead.

- **Stock up.** Watch for sales on organic frozen produce; when you find a bargain, stock up!

12

By the Way,
This Is Spiritual...

As a Christian, I can't complete this book without adding my personal, spiritual convictions to all the medical and scientific arguments for a healthy change in lifestyle. I believe God takes a huge interest in what we put into our bodies. After all, the Bible is full of references to food, dating back to the very beginning of our existence. But the matter, again, isn't just about physically ingesting food; it is a matter of attitude, conscience, and stewardship. And sometimes, those can be bigger obstacles than what exists in the physical realm.

Recall Matthew 26:41: "Watch and pray, that ye enter not into temptation: the spirit indeed *is* willing but the flesh *is* weak."

Granted, in this Scripture, Jesus was referring to His disciples' ability to pray for a length of time, but the principle still applies. Our spirit always wants to do better than our flesh is inclined to do. The challenge is always to keep our flesh in a vigilant state that follows what our spirit *already knows* is the right thing to do.

The Sleeping Church

I want to introduce a different perspective. Have you ever overeaten at a holiday? About three hours after such an elaborate meal, many of us feel ready for a nap. And, if it is indeed a holiday, it may be one of only a couple days out of the year that we give ourselves "permission" to overeat." What if, a few hours after a huge holiday meal, you had to stand and fight, ready for battle? Would you be physically fit to do so? If you knew that morning that this activity would be required of you, would you eat differently at the table?

I believe Christians all over the world are beginning to feel that we are on the edge of a great spiritual awakening, a time of potentially massive, worldwide revival and radical spreading of the Gospel of Jesus Christ. If this is true, what would be the most effective way to render the Body of Christ ineffective? By rendering *individuals* within the church unproductive. And how are we made fruitless? Through distraction, illness, and fatigue. When it comes to our food, many of us, though we may be aware that there is a problem, are overwhelmed, confused, and unsure of where to even begin find out what's wrong and come up with solutions that would lead us to better health.

What better way to thwart a spiritual awakening than by making sure that everyone is sick, tired, and distracted?

When Moses sent Israelites out to investigate the Promised Land, he sent them out with a list of specific questions they were to come back able to answer (see Numbers 13 and 14). Moses wasn't looking for *emotions*—he didn't need to know how they felt about the land; rather, Moses was looking for *information*. He wanted to know specifics about what they found there. But they returned with statements based on their emotions: They were afraid, they felt powerless, and they were uncertain about how to proceed.

The Israelites even went so far as to make the following statement to Moses and Aaron: "If only we had died in Egypt! Or in this wilderness!

Why is the Lord bringing us to this land only to let us fall by the sword? Our wives and children will be taken as plunder. Wouldn't it be better for us to go back to Egypt?" God punished this wildly emotional response by refusing to allow their generation to see the Promised Land.

This may seem like an extreme circumstance to compare with our current attitude about improving our diets. I'm not saying that our complacency toward our food matches this scenario in its rebellious intensity. I *am* saying that when we arrive at a place where we are unsure of our path or are afraid to proceed, emotions such as fear and uncertainty aren't righteous reasons to neglect action. God doesn't want us to stall out in our insecurity, and He certainly doesn't want us standing around powerless, simply "going with the flow." Like the Israelites, we cannot embrace complacency simply because we *feel* afraid, powerless, and uncertain of how to proceed. We must collect information, setting our emotions aside. This is when the plan of action will begin to surface, and we can stand, awake and ready to follow the course ahead.

As I mentioned earlier, a current increase in spiritual activity appears to be leading toward an awakening. We must be effective, which requires setting emotional or fearful responses aside and determining a strategic course of action.

Surrendering That First Ingredient

We must likewise be wary of the enemy's appeal to our own human reasoning. Second Corinthians 10:5, which says, "Casting down imaginations, and every high thing that exalteth itself against the knowledge of God, and bringing into captivity every thought to the obedience of Christ," demands that we bring *every* thought under the submission of God's will for our lives. Then we must remember that when we know there is something we *should* do, we must not try to "reason" our way out of doing it.

Consider the snake in the Garden of Eden as tempted Eve. Scripture shows that even this first sin of mankind was accomplished because of the serpent's appeal to the human ability to reason and, ironically, that temptation was presented using food. Granted, I want to be very clear that the real sin was *disobedience to God*, but the *tools* used by the enemy were the vehicles of *our own thought process* and *food*. If the serpent had approached Eve with a weapon, for example, this story may have ended differently. The snake's approach was subtle.

By surrendering that first toxic ingredient in our food—our attitude toward it—we place ourselves in a state of willingness to follow God's will in our lives and make the changes that He asks us to make.

We're under Attack

I will wager that the decline in our food industry and eating habits over the last hundred years is a type of Trojan horse: a "sleeper" method of attack on humanity. It is only the latest onslaught in a continued attack on creation that dates all the way back to the beginning of the world. Bold statement? Absolutely. But bear with me as I make my case.

As shown through the story of the first sin of mankind, God has placed limits on what we should eat. Adam and Eve were instructed about what was forbidden: "And the Lord God commanded the man saying, Of every tree of the garden thou mayest freely eat: But of the tree of the knowledge of good and evil, thou shall not eat of it: for in the day that thou eatest thereof thou shalt surely die" (Genesis 2:16–17). Then, after the first couple was cast out of the garden for the sin of breaking that one rule, God changed our relationship with food as part of our punishment: "Thorns also and thistles shall bring forth to thee; and thou shalt eat the herb of the field; In the sweat of thy face shalt thou eat bread, till thou return on to the ground" (Genesis 3:18–19).

To repeat: I'm not saying that the disobedience in the Garden of

Eden was merely about food. The first sin concerned obedience to God and following His instructions. When man sinned, however, our relationship to food changed, as recorded in the Scripture above. Like so many other aspects of creation, it had been given to us in the beginning as a pleasurable aspect of life. And, *like so many other aspects of creation*, that changed when man fell, and food is now being used against mankind.

Throughout the rest of the Bible, there are many other references to food. Because our relationship to food changed at the Fall and has continued to evolve over the centuries, what was originally intended to be life-sustaining and healthy has become toxic and dangerous. As stated previously, what should be friend has become, in many ways, foe. And, like so many other threats we face today, even if we're aware of the problem, we often find ourselves frozen in place, unsure of how to proceed. Most of us feel powerless, uneducated, confused about where to begin, and generally insecure. At the core of this paralysis lies our lack of knowledge, motivation, and empowerment.

Lack of Knowledge Will Destroy Us

My people are destroyed for lack of knowledge. (Hosea 4:6)

We live in the age of knowledge. Never has a generation enjoyed freer access to more education, research, news, technology, and other information than the present one. Many homes have more than one computer, and a simple Internet search engine can tell us nearly anything we want to know. Books abound, free tutorials and online classes are everywhere, and do-it-yourself TV shows are available on nearly every channel. Knowledge is all around us, although it may seem hidden at times. We must work, discipline, and educate ourselves to keep from being destroyed by the enemy. This is one way we Christians should seize every opportunity to be vigilant.

The reason God the Father imposed the first rule on man, though presented in the form of a dietary limitation, was that, from the very start, He knew some things we put into our *physical* bodies present a danger far beyond the physical realm. By committing the disobedient act of eating the forbidden fruit, we placed our spiritual condition at risk.

A deeper truth that dates back as far as the origin of mankind and is also evident in the events in the Garden of Eden is the ongoing, ever-present enemy attack. Creation has always been under some kind of assault since the very beginning, and our current time is no exception. We see by the events leading up to the Flood in Genesis that man's flesh was under attack at that time. God intervened, and man was rescued from this attack. But over the ages, the onslaught continues. Each time God intervenes and man changes his behavior, the enemy recoils and comes up with a new, sneakier type of assault. Christians must be watchful.

Think of all the gifts God gave us that are now corrupt because we haven't enjoyed them within His guidelines or as He intended. A few examples are Christian fellowship, sex, financial prosperity, and relationships. Even the innate, childlike innocence of our kids is corrupted by images bombarding our children from the media they encounter each day through no control or intention of their own: billboards, TV programs and commercials, and certain conversations heard in public and even in their homes! Each time we become wise to the attack that we are facing and learn to combat it, we must be wary of a new tactic that will soon appear.

What better way to fight an enemy than by "getting inside his head?" And, if this method doesn't work, a natural subsequent tactic by the enemy would be to try to weaken us physically to make us too sick and tired to fight. Think of a parent who has many small children running all about the house, creating chaos. We may envision that person being "beaten into submission," too tired to effectively care for the children, allowing the chaos to escalate because he or she simply doesn't have the energy to stand his or her ground anymore. This helpless, outnumbered feeling is not unlike the resignation we might feel about spiritual matters when we are fighting a battle that keeps us fatigued, sick, or even dying. This can be a much more effective strategy than an overt attack that we recognize and meet with resistance.

Understanding how excitotoxins cross our blood-brain barrier and impact our mind *through our hormonal glands*, the theories on the numerous ways this could affect our thought processes could be speculated upon forever. Because our hormones are indirectly under a type of attack, this could be having an impact on sexual immorality, impulse control, or even gender issues. At the very least, our judgment is impaired by the constant chemical onslaught our minds are suffering. And when we are *conditioned* to this, we don't even realize we're off track. The enemy could win a battle we don't even realize we're fighting! If you think this is a stretch, consider trying to reason with an intoxicated man. His thoughts *truly make sense to him* in the heat of an argument. Because he is under the influence of an alcoholic substance, he can't even see that his thought process is irrational. If we're under the influence of mind-altering chemicals such as those found in many foods, we're leaving our entire judgment process vulnerable to the influence of disreputable sources. Unless we detox, open our eyes, and ask God to give us discernment and help us develop the mind of Christ, we have left our discernment compromised. Adding to this the connection between the gut and the brain, it becomes obvious that our brain—the "control center"—is truly under attack.

The Gut-Mind Connection
Goes Back to the Beginning

In the Old Testament, the Bible says that Joseph, after years of hardship, "Lifted up his eyes, and saw his brother Benjamin, his mother's son, and said, Is this your younger brother, of whom ye spake unto me? And he said, God be gracious unto the, my son. And Joseph made haste; for his bowels did yearn upon his brother: and he sought where to weep; and he entered into his chamber, and wept there" (Genesis 43:29–30). Notice that the Scripture said his *bowels* yearned. References like this are found throughout the Bible. Modern science reveals the connection between the mind and the gut by explaining that millions of nerves link the gut directly to the brain. We also now know about how many of the ingredients in the foods we eat can cross the blood-brain barrier, affecting the brain as well. But think about this: The relationship between the mind and the gut is such an innate knowledge held by each of us that it is integrated in the *simple daily language we use*. For example, if I'm certain something will go right, I might say, "I've got a gut feeling about this." Or another example might be on a day that I get really bad news, I might say, "That hit me right in the gut." When children are angry, one of the first insults they learn to say to each other is, "I hate your guts," which is like saying, "I hate you to the core of your being." The list goes on. We use many phrases about our "guts" on a daily basis without even thinking about it.

Recall the woman described in 1 Kings 3:26 who was willing to give her child to another woman to save her baby's life: "Then spake the woman whose living child was on to the King, for her bowels yearned upon her son."

Or consider Philemon 1:7, which says, "For we have great joy and consolation in my love, because the bowels of the saints are refreshed by thee, brother."

My point in bringing up these Scriptures is to illustrate that the guts and the mind have been associated since the beginning of time. What is felt within the center of the body—the guts—has always immediately been presumed to be connected with the spirit: emotions, patterns, and overall individual dedication. This means that beyond all the other arguments made in this book, on a spiritual level, when we aren't eating well, we are placing our core thought-processing unit in a vulnerable place, and could be compromising our very ability to think clearly and make good, righteous decisions in our everyday lives.

So, understanding that even on a scriptural level there *is* a connection between the mind and the gut, coupled with the knowledge that there is a scientific base for that belief as well, it stands to reason that by vetting what we are eating, we are safeguarding our *thought process*, our *sound judgment*, and thereby even our *ability to fully serve God*. (Note: My dear friend Pastor Caspar McCloud, in his book entitled *What Was I Thinking?*, has written drawn some of the most profound conclusions I've ever read on the power of thoughts and their ability to influence our physical and spiritual health.)

Your Body Is the Temple

I'm sure that if you have attended church, you've at some point heard this Scripture: "What? know ye not that your body is the temple of the Holy Ghost which is in you, which ye have of God, and ye are not your own? For ye are bought with a price: therefore glorify God in your body, and in your spirit, which are God's" (1 Corinthians 6:19–20).

When you encountered this passage in church, the context used was likely to make an argument against drinking, smoking, or fornication; but I imagine you probably never heard it used regarding food. But if we *know* that by indulging in unhealthy eating habits, we are placing our health and judgment in harm's way, that activity should fall also under the jurisdiction of this Scripture, shouldn't it? I'm not talking about beating ourselves up over what we've done to our bodies in the past; but as it pertains to the *future*, I ask: If we *knowingly* overeat, allowing obesity, chronic illness, heart disease, or other health impairments to stack up within our bodies, are we in a position to judge someone who is drinking or smoking?

God Wants Us to Be Good Stewards

Titus 2:7 says, "In all things shewing thyself a pattern of good works: in doctrine shewing on corruption us, gravity, sincerity, sound speech, that cannot be condemned."

Many Scriptures speak of important principles like being good stewards, being trustworthy, and not being overindulgent or "given to excess." Why shouldn't these principles apply to our food as well? I believe God has strong opinions about our eating habits.

The parable of the steward in Matthew chapter 25 documents the story of three servants who were entrusted with their master's property during his absence. When the master returned, he required an accounting from the servants of how they had handled his property while he had been away. You may know how the story ends: Two servants were deemed wise in the way they handled the property; the other was not. The two wise servants were celebrated and the third was called wicked and slothful—or, in some translations of the Bible, lazy.

I want to be very clear that I'm not saying that sick people are wicked or lazy. Likewise, I'm *not* stating that a person with diabetes, cancer, or other chronic illness is being punished for sin, wickedness, or laziness. I *am* saying that *anything* we have been entrusted with is something we'll eventually have to account for. If we can avoid disease and take care of our bodies, we'll have more years to remain here on earth to work in God's service. A person who can take steps to remain healthy and add years to his or her life will parallel the servant who was left with five talents and returned with ten on the day of accounting. An individual who can increase his or her life for any length of time in order to further a God-ordained commission is similar to the servant who returned with more talents than he or she was originally entrusted with.

Jesus' Miracles Involved Food and Drinks

In Matthew 14, Jesus took five loaves and two fish and fed an entire multitude, which included about five thousand men *besides* the uncounted women and children. At the end of the seaside supper, there were twelve full baskets of bread and fish left. When it appeared that there were more people than there was food to feed them, Jesus could've sent the crowd away, but He did not. He chose to *feed* them. He could've given them *just enough,* but he chose to make more than enough.

Or, consider the first miracle that Jesus performed, discussed in John chapter 2:10: "And saith unto him, Every man at the beginning doth set forth good wine; and when men have well drunk, then that which is worse: but thou hast kept the good wine until now."

While this was not a miracle involving *food*, it did provide something for human consumption. Judging by the comment in the verse, at this point in the wedding, *any* wine would have been sufficient. But that isn't what Jesus provided. He made a *superior product.* There is a point in these observations. I believe food is important to God, but I also believe that He wants us to do the best job that we can with our food, not only in quantity, but in quality as well.

God Condemns Gluttony

On the other side of the spectrum, God condemns gluttony: Whose end is destruction, whose God is their belly, and whose glory is in their shame, who mind earthly things. (Philippians 3:19)

For everything in the world—the lust of the flesh, the lust of the eyes, and the pride of life—comes not from the father but from the world. (1 John 2:16)

For the drunkard and the glutton shall come to poverty: and drowsiness shall clothe a man with rags. (Proverbs 23:21)

The above passages are only a few of many that talk about us not being given to our fleshly desires, but transcending to a place where we look to *Him* to meet our needs. The desires of the flesh are often misconstrued as being merely sexual, but this isn't always true. The desires of the flesh include anything finite that keeps us from following the will of God. When we are fatigued, sluggish, or ineffective, our discernment cannot be sharpened. To truly surrender to the will of God is to follow Him in *all* our ways. Especially in light of the knowledge that many of us are biologically addicted to food, this heightens the alarm that our food is a combatant that we must arm ourselves against.

Be IN the World, But Not of It

Let's be honest: Changing a diet is hard. It is especially difficult in our modern economy, with our rat-race schedules and the lack of healthy food that's available. But the Bible never guarantees that following God's orders is be easy. Perhaps another way of being "in this world, but not of this world" is by taking the harder route, forsaking pleasures of the flesh (seduction of food, especially with flavor enhancers and biologically addictive ingredients) and following the route we know is healthiest and safest, even though it is difficult: "Enter ye in at the strait gate: for wide is the gate, and broad is the way, that leadeth to destruction, and many there be which go in thereat: because strait is the gate, and narrow is the way, which leadeath unto life, and few there be that find it," (Matthew 7:13–14).

If a verse were ever designed to describe the selection at a grocery store, this is it. "Broad" are the aisles that lead to junk foods, excitotoxins, flavor enhancers, GMOs, and so much more destruction. Very, *very* "narrow," if there is one at all, is the aisle that leads to whole, safe, organic foods. But, like in the rest of our journey, God does not promise us this will be easy. In fact, we've been guaranteed that it will probably be very hard at times. But this is how we prove ourselves, and this is how we grow. This is how we learn to die to our flesh and choose God's will above our own. Through these experiences, not only will we learn, we will be able to guide others, and the discipline of surrendering our fleshly desires becomes easier each time we practice it.

God Expects Us to Fast

"Therefore also now," saith the Lord, "turn ye even to me with all your heart, with fasting, and weeping, and with mourning." (Joel 2:12)

Moreover when ye fast, be not, as the hypocrites, of a sad countenance: for they disfigure their faces, that they may appear unto men to fast. Verily I say unto you, they have their reward. (Matthew 6:16)

As you may already have noted, the second passage listed above says *when* you fast, not *if* you fast.

Consider Donald S. Whitney's statement on fasting from his work, *Spiritual Disciplines for the Christian Life*: "Christians in a gluttonous, denial-less, self-indulgent society may struggle to accept and begin the practice of fasting. Few Disciplines go so radically against the flesh and the mainstream of culture as this one. Nevertheless, we dare not overlook its biblical significance."[181]

Whitney goes on to explain that fasting should be connected to a spiritual purpose. He outlines a real-life scenario something like this: "As you are fasting and your head aches or your stomach growls and you think, *I'm hungry!* your next thought is likely to be something like, *Oh, right—I'm hungry because I'm fasting today.* Then your next thought *should* be, *And I'm fasting for this purpose:* [insert spiritual reason here.]"[182]

The spiritual motivation behind the fast should be what comes to mind when the hunger reminds you that you haven't eaten. Each time we're reminded of the hunger we're reminded us to pray. Perhaps you have had trouble with 1 Thessalonians 5:17, which says we should "pray without ceasing." Going without food and having the constant hunger remind us to pray might help us learn how to follow this scriptural command.

Arthur Wallis, in his work, *God's Chosen Fast,* spoke of how fasting can heighten the determination of our prayer:

> Fasting is calculated to bring a note of urgency and importunity to our praying, and to give force to our pleading in the court of heaven. The man who prays with fasting is giving heaven notice that he is truly in earnest.… He is using a means that God has chosen to make his voice be heard on high.[183]

Fasts are also effective when a group or nation wants to seek communal prayer. In the book of Jonah, the king of Nineveh called for a nationwide fast as a show of repentance:

> So the people of Nineveh believed God, and proclaimed a fast, and put on sackcloth, from the greatest of them even to the least of them. For word came unto the king of Nineveh, and he arose from his throne, and he laid his robe from him, and covered him with sackcloth, and set in ashes. And he caused it to be proclaimed and published through Nineveh by decree of the

king and his nobles, saying, Let neither man nor beast, heard nor flock, taste anything: let them not feed, nor drink water. But let man and beast be covered with sackcloth, and cry mightily unto God: yea, let them turn every one from his evil way, and from the violence that is in their hands. Who can tell if God will turn and repent, and turn away from his fierce anger, that we perish not? And God saw their works, that they turned from their evil way; and God repented of the evil, that he had said that he would do unto them; and he did it not. (Jonah 3:5–10)

Beyond all the spiritual applications of fasting, there are physical benefits as well. CNBC Online recently released an article about a diet program that will soon be released for sale. The benefits cited about the concept of fasting are worth noting:

The research Institute also put rodents on a fast-mimicking diet twice a month for four days. At the end of each FMD [fast-mimicking diet] period, blood glucose levels were 40 percent lower, a finding the study's authors suggest may show that fasting can help with diabetes and other degenerative diseases. The results, published in Cell, noted that the mice, even after returned to a regular diet and biological readings, still had less tumors, inflammation and other health issues associated with age.[184]

Another study, this time involving seventy-one people, showed that those who practiced a diet involving fasting decreased the production of IGF-1, a hormone within the body that contributes to aging and disease.[185] Subjects also showed a reduction in C-reactive protein, which has been linked to general inflammation and a variety of other diseases like heart disease or cancer.

God Wants Us to Be Vigilant

Be sober, be vigilant; because your adversary the devil, as a roaring lion, walketh about, seeking whom he may devour. (1 Peter 5:8)

Continue in prayer, and watch in the same with thanksgiving. (Colossians 4:2)

These Scriptures charge us to be vigilant. I cannot recall a place in the Bible that tells believers to go to sleep, bury their heads in the sand, or simply wait until things get better. God is always encouraging His people to take action. We are always to be watchful and ready to act when necessary. Further, we're to share the knowledge we gain with the upcoming generations: "Only give heed to thyself, and keep thy soul diligently, lest thou forget the things which thine eyes have seen, and lest they depart from thy heart all the days of thy life; but teach them thy sons, and thy sons' sons" (Deuteronomy 4:9).

The damage we've done to our bodies in our ignorance of threat can largely be reversed if we will make the necessary changes. More importantly, we can reach out and help those in need to find their way in the knowledge that we have shared. Like everything else addressed to the Church, it's important that we not go back to sleep in the light of new information. It is up to the church to stand, be vigilant, and be activists.

Important Events Have Happened over Food

As stated previously, God has intervened in the matters involving food since the beginning of the human race. In the book of Exodus, it's recorded that He caused manna to appear on the ground each day:

And when the dew that lay was gone up, behold, upon the face of the wilderness there lay a small round thing, as small as the hoar frost on the ground. And when the children of Israel saw it, they said to one another, It is manna: for they wist not what it was. And Moses said unto them, This is the bread which the Lord hath given you to eat. (Exodus 16:14–15)

Also recall the incident recorded in 1 Kings 17, when Elijah was told to flee to Cherith. He was told to drink from the brook, and God commanded the ravens to deliver a meal of "bread and flesh" twice each day. The Bible doesn't tell us that God elaborated on other orders for Elijah. It does not say that God gave him instructions on what he might wear, what kind of bedding he might use, or whether he was supposed to take a weapon to defend himself. He was simply told to hide for time, but, hand in hand with that order, God saw to the provision of his *immediate needs*, the top priority about which appear to be consumption. This indicates that God places a high-priority marker on what we eat and drink. He could have just as easily set Elijah's physiological system not to *need* to eat or drink during that period of time. But that isn't what happened. Not only did God Himself see to Elijah's physical needs, but He involved other elements of creation—ravens and the brook—to meet those needs. Later in the same chapter of 1 Kings, another miracle of food occurred when Elijah encountered a widow who was preparing to eat her last meal with her son. When Elijah asked her to share her meal, she told him she did not have enough. The subsequent miracle was initiated by an act of sacrificial obedience on the part of the widow: "And Elijah said unto her, Fear not; go and do as thou hast said: but make me thereof a little cake first, and bring *it* unto me, and after make for the and for thy son" (1 Kings 17:13). The widow obeyed Elijah's orders, and she and her household ate for "…many days. And the barrel of meal wasted not, neither did the cruse of oil fail, according to the word of the Lord" (1 Kings 17:15–16). The woman's willingness to obey, even at the risk of dire consequences (possibly giving the last food available to a stranger instead of feeding her own son), placed herself and her son within the path of blessing.

An interesting comparison can be observed in Matthew 7:9–10, "Or what man is there of you, whom if his son ask bread, will he give him a stone? Or if he ask a fish, will he give him a serpent?" This Scripture isn't talking about food, but about prayer and our relationship with God. However, it's worth noting that Jesus used a comparison of us feeding our children.

Jesus Used Food and Wine to Represent His Body as a Sacrifice

The statement for biblical comparison regarding food wouldn't be complete if we didn't note that Jesus used bread and wine to represent His sacrifice on the cross. Jesus had arranged to have supper with the Twelve:

> And as they were eating, Jesus took bread, and blessed it, and brake it, and gave it to the disciples, and said, Take, eat; this is my body. And he took the cup, and gave thanks, and gave it to them, saying, Drink ye all of it; for this is my blood of the new testament, which is shed for many for the remission of sins. But I say unto you, I will not drink henceforth of this fruit of the vine, until that day when I drink it new with you in my father's kingdom. (Matthew 26:26–29)

A lot's going on in this passage. First of all, Jesus, the Bread of Life, instructs the Twelve to eat the bread to remember that His body is broken for them. Jesus is the fulfillment, the sustenance, of all we need. Then, He instructs the men around the table to drink the wine, which represents the blood He would soon spill to take away the sin of man. This represents the salvation plan and all God has done to show His immense love for us, despite our lack of worthiness. Jesus then promises that He will not drink of the fruit of the vine until He is with these men again, in His Father's kingdom. He explains the sacrifice He is about to make, although the Twelve cannot yet comprehend what He is saying. He promises that after He makes His sacrifice, they will be together in heaven. All these amazing promises and gifts to man for all time were relayed to the disciples by Jesus Himself, using food and drink.

God Ministers through Food

Furthermore, the outreach of food is important to God. We see Jesus' instructions in Luke 14:12–14:

> Then said he also to him that bade him, When thou makest a dinner or a supper, call not thy friends, nor thy brethren, neither thy kinsman, nor thy rich neighbours; lest they also bid the again, and a recompense be made thee. But when thou makest a feast, call the poor, the maimed, the lame, the blind: and thou shalt be blessed; for they cannot recompense thee: for thou shalt be recompensed at the resurrection of the just.

Food is so important to God that is one of the needs we're ordered to meet as Christians. Recall the story of the sheep and the goats:

> When the Son of man shall come in his glory, and all the holy angels with him, then shall he sit upon the throne of his glory: and before him shall be gathered all nations: and he shall

separate them one from another, as a shepherd divideth his sheep from the goats:… Then shall the King say unto them.… Come, ye blessed of my Father, inherit the kingdom prepared for you from the foundation of the world: for I was hungered, and ye gave me meat: I was thirsty, and ye gave me drink.… Then shall the righteous answer him, saying, Lord, when saw we thee and hungered, and fed thee?... And the King shall answer and say unto them, Verily I say unto you, Inasmuch as ye have done it unto the least of my brethren, ye have done it unto me. (Matthew 25:31–45)

The reader probably knows the rest of the story, wherein God addresses the people who *did not* meet the physical needs of those they encountered throughout their lives. Granted, this Scripture tackles much more than food. It discusses clothing, shelter, sick or elderly visitation, and more. For the purpose of this book, I'm only emphasizing the part that refers to food. But, the bottom line remains: God holds food in a high priority where ministry and outreach are concerned, and this order is simply too profound to disregard. If you are one of the blessed 20 percent of people in this country who are not suffering from the symptoms outlined throughout this book, surely you know someone who *is*. There are sick people in the world right now who feel powerless to take control of their situations, and *you* can be poised to help them if you will only take what you've learned from this book and reach out to them.

God Promises a Feast in Heaven

Beyond the fact that food is a recurring theme throughout Scripture passages that address physical life on earth, many refer to food as part of our future in eternity with God:

And in this mountain shall the Lord of hosts make unto all people a feast of fat things, a feast of wines on the lees, of fat things in full of marrow, of wines on the lees well refined. (Isaiah 25:6)

And I appoint unto you a kingdom, as my father hath appointed unto me; that ye may eat and drink at my table in my kingdom, and sit on thrones judging the 12 tribes of Israel. (Luke 22:29–30)

And I say unto you, That many shall come from the East and West, and shall sit down with Abraham, and Isaac, and Jacob, in the kingdom of heaven. (Matthew 8:11)

And he saith unto me, Write, Blessed are they which are called on to the marriage supper of the Lamb. And he saith unto me, These are the true sayings of God. (Revelation 19:9)

Because they believed not in God, entrusted not in his salvation: though he had commanded the clouds from above, and opened the doors of heaven, and had rained down manna upon them to eat, and had given them the corn of heaven. Man did eat angels' food: he sent them meat to the full. (Psalm 78:22–25)

If food is so important to God that He plans to include it in our spiritual existence with Him in heaven, then surely we must prove ourselves worthy by taking care of how we handle it in this life.

My Nightly Prayer

In addition to now taking full responsibility over everything my family puts into or on their bodies, and being as proactive as I know how to be, eradicating all chemicals from our home, I now say a prayer over my family every night. I pray for each member of my entire extended family. I pray from the top of their heads to the bottom of their feet that every cell is commanded to be regenerated in perfect health. I pray against cancer and disease, bacteria and viruses, and infections. I pray that God will forgive us for any unknown damages we may have contributed to through food chemicals, vaccines, or other chemical exposure we have allowed into our bodies and those of our children. I pray that God will pardon my children from any physical consequences that may have derived from my total lack of knowledge during previous years about what we were feeding them, and that He would free my children from any damages caused by anything they ate because of the ignorance of their parents. I pray that every organ in their bodies will function perfectly, and that their hypothalamus glands will be healthy and send healing signals to their bodies wherever needed. I also pray that they will fully receive the nutrients of our efforts, both physically and spiritually. I ask God to bolster their immune system and prevent sediment from settling in their organs, and that their bodies will be purged of iniquity. I pray that they will hormonally, spiritually, and nutritionally receive what they need, and not suffer emotionally or mentally because of food they've eaten. We anoint them with anointing olive oil at the first sight of fever, sickness, or infection. Then I pray about their futures, for their future spouses, and that as parents we will have the wisdom to guide them each day. I pray that the children will grow up with a zeal to serve Him. I also pray for the prodigal children of several of our dearest friends and for their health, along with the constantly evolving needs and matters of intervention that life brings. I also whisper God's praise over my family and thank Him for His many abundant blessings, and all the evidence that He's at work in our lives constantly. This may sound like an unusual prayer, but I pray it every night.

My prayer for you is that you will find health and maintain it. I pray you have found tools in this book that you need to take charge of your health and find a true path of healing, as I have done. But most of all, my prayer is that you know Jesus as your personal Lord and Savior, and that your continued path with Him will bring you all that you need in this life.

13

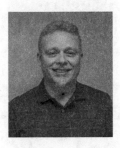

Dr. Matthew Sams,
DC, FIACA

Have you ever noticed that some of the greatest journeys to discovery in our lives can be traced back to a time of great pain, tragedy, or seeming uncertainty? A time when we feel hopeless, powerless, or lost? A time when we are searching for truth, wisdom, or even just a glimmer of hope? This feeling inside of us that there must be something more? There must be something different! My journey into natural medicine began this same way!

I was born in 1970 in rural Iowa—the son of a heavy equipment contractor and a factory worker. My parents were hard workers. You had to be desperately sick in those days, at least with my family, to merit a trip to the doctor. Of the three doctors in our farming town, my parents took me to a doctor reminiscent of ol' Doc Baker from the *Little House on the Prairie* TV show. Though he may have carried a black leather bag and made house calls in earlier years, by the time I can remember seeing him, he was pretty old. I am confident that he saw patients whether they had two legs or four. Every person who saw him, regardless of the reason, received at least two things: 1) a shot of penicillin in the arm and 2) a manila envelope of various sulfa pills to take.

One time around 1982, when I was 12 years old, I had a sickness that I just could not shake. After dealing with it for about two weeks, my parents finally took me to Ol' Doc Baker. Sure enough, I got my shot and my envelope of pills. For whatever reason, this time was different. I remember waking up early that next morning needing to go to the bathroom. My mom was already up, getting ready to go to work at the factory. I stood there at the bathroom, and then the lights went out.

My mom heard me hit the ground and ran to wake up my dad. They dialed up Doc Baker, and were told, "We cannot handle that kind of thing here. You need to get him to Des Moines as fast as you can." By then, I had regained consciousness. My parents loaded me into the Impala, and Dad shortened that one-hour drive to about thirty minutes. To this day, I remember looking up at the speedometer needle being buried far past the numbers on the display.

As we entered the hospital in Des Moines, this began my own personal Damascus Road experience. I was immediately admitted into the hospital and they began treating me for an extreme allergic reaction to sulfa drugs (the ones in the manila envelope). Though it is easy for me to remember, it is hard for me to put into words. I remember lying there in the hospital bed. I remember what everything looked like. I remember seeing the *shekinah* glory of the Lord. I remember this concept being put on my heart: "This isn't it." I remember it all so vividly, yet to put this experience into words that you could understand—I cannot! Just to say, like any encounter someone has with the Most High God, these people leave marked or different. Just as happened with Abraham, Jacob, Isaac, Moses, Stephen, Paul, John and others, when God revealed Himself to me that day in the hospital, I would never be the same again. This encounter made me into the person I am today!

What "wasn't it," you may ask? "IT" was these things: that style of Western medicine and how I was being treated for my sickness; the "take two of these (drugs) and call me in the morning" mentality; and the "treat everything with a shot and a pill" concept. This revelation in my life that "this wasn't it" created a life-long and insatiable appetite in me for knowledge. At this point, I began to question everything. In fact, my vision statement that we have for our office is to "Question the Status Quo" in everything we do. I began realizing that for too long people had been treating symptoms and not the causes.

As soon as I was well enough to get out of the house, I spent countless hours at the library. Keep in mind that these were the days before search engines and the Internet. These were the days of books. I would bypass the card catalog at the library and head to the nonfiction section 610: Medicine & Health. I would walk down the aisles of that section and read the titles of those books. If a title interested me, I would read that book or sections of it that had information I wanted to learn. I looked up articles on microfilm to read and gain knowledge of how the body worked. I became a student of the body, how it worked, and why it worked. This remains a study pursuit that I will not graduate from until the day I die.

A couple of years later, my mother was in an automobile accident and began to see a chiropractor in town. Mom would finish her day at the factory and I would finish my day at school around the same time. We would meet at this chiropractor's office, and I would observe Mom getting treatments for her injuries. At this point, I knew chiropractic care was part of my journey. Even after Mom finished her treatments, I would shadow this doctor almost every day after school. He discipled me in the art of chiropractic medicine. He took me under his wing, showed me what he knew, and answered my many questions—or at least told me where to go look up the answers. When I was a senior in high school, the doctor drove me the four hours to his alma mater, Palmer Chiropractic College, for a college visit. He was adamant that this was where I needed to attend.

During my undergraduate studies at Iowa State, God directed me to another chiropractor who also mentored and showed me the importance of whole food supplements. Food is medicine; it's no different than how food can be poison. Logically, if what you ingest can make you ill, could what you ingest make you better, too? This doctor and I would go to seminars, conferences, and workshops. We would always be learning. This is key! By the time I was graduating from chiropractic college, I was also teaching an elective class for the college in a new method of chiropractic adjusting I had learned about and studied.

After graduation, I was hired by my second mentor. He began to study a concept called acupuncture that has been around for thousands of years. He really wanted me to learn it with him. I, however, had a check in my spirit about this. Though I did not grow up in church all my life, I am the grandson of a preacher, and my family had begun actively attending church just prior to my Damascus Road experience. I had given my life to Christ as a 10-year-old boy prior to my encounter with God. I saw acupuncture as a form of voodoo. How could punctures to the skin make one better? I wrestled with this concept for many weeks and finally broke down and set up an appointment with my pastor.

During my two-hour visit with him, I was the only one talking. I laid out to him what acupuncture was; the history of acupuncture; how it could help a person; how it could be misperceived; and how I did not want to be viewed as doing something that was against God. After I finished, the pastor looked up and said, "What are YOU going to do with acupuncture? Are you intending it for good or for evil?" Then he was silent again. I told him that anything I do, I want to do for good and never for evil.

It was this meeting, after a great wrestling match with God, that I realized this simple truth—HEALING IS (AND ALWAYS WILL

BE) GOD'S. If other cultures have perverted that simple truth, they are stealing something that is God's. Because God created the body to heal and created the plants for food, with my practice, I will just go into the enemy's camp and take back what he has stolen from us to begin with! By the way, that pastor quickly became one of my patients after I received my certification.

Over the past nineteen years of practicing on my own, we have developed somewhat of a following at our office. It is not uncommon on a weekly basis for people to drive more than four hours each way to receive treatment and consultation at our practice. We have some who fly in to visit our practice. A common question from these sojourners is: Where can I find a doctor near me who can help me in this journey away from constant prescriptions, patches, and probes, a doctor who will not just keep giving me chemical after chemical to put in my body? This is a complicated answer and a potentially long journey, but a worthwhile one.

Maybe this is where you are in your journey. If you're asking yourself, "How do I find a natural medicine practitioner?" First, let us start with some basics:

1) **SET REALISTIC EXPECTATIONS:** In alternative or mainstream medicine, there is no such thing as "one size fits all." Just like with your family practice doctor, you cannot expect any one person to have all the answers. This is the reason for specialists. I would not want a plastic surgeon performing open heart surgery on me. That is not what they do. When finding an alternative medicine, natural medicine, functional medicine, or other non-mainstream health provider, do not put unrealistic expectations on them Do not expect them to fix in one visit what you created in a lifetime.

2) **IT IS NOT CHEAP:** This road-less-traveled journey you are on is one that often is not covered by insurance. Often the whole-food supplements and nutraceuticals that you will take are not available in the $4 generic section of the local superstore.

That being said, do not let yourself be taken advantage of! At our office, we treat every person as a unique and individual case. I cannot tell patients that they will get better in "X" number of visits, because each body is different. We have had patients who have gotten better almost instantly and some who are peeling back their body issues one layer at a time like the layers of an onion. Beware of "package" deals that stipulate a certain number of visits for a large amount of money up front. What if your body responds faster or slower than the "package"? What if you need an entirely different type of treatment that is not offered in that clinic, but you do not find out until mid-way through your "package deal"?

3) **QUALITY DOES MATTER:** I am a firm believer in feeding your body the proper nutrients it needs to survive and thrive. Just because you can buy a cheaper version of something with the same name as a product recommended by an alternative medicine provider does not mean that it will have the same efficacy as the product your provider recommends.

Using omega-3 oil as an example, we have had multiple patients come into our office with stomach issues. After getting a thorough understanding of what vitamins and supplements they were taking, we discovered that they were taking an omega-3 oil as a preventative for heart issues. They had purchased this omega-3 in bulk from a wholesale club or big box store. By simply switching them to a properly manufactured, quality omega-3, their stomach issues subsided. The quality of the product you are putting in your body matters, from the grocery store to the health food store.

4) **ARE THEY LIFELONG LEARNERS?** That day I spent in the hospital as a child, I began my journey of learning. I have always want to be learning. Technology is changing. New discoveries are being made. If practitioners you are seeing stopped learning

new things the day they got their degree, they are probably not the best people to be seeing. The knowledge being gained in the healthcare profession is very similar to cell phones and computers. It becomes outdated quickly.

5) **DR. GOOGLE, MD:** I read one time a quote from Abraham Lincoln that says, "You can't trust everything you read on the internet." For every type of test, every type of doctor, every type of mainstream treatment, and every type of alternative treatment, I can find a web page that is either in favor of or against those things. Do your research from reputable sources. You cannot trust everything you read on the Internet.

6) **THREATENED BY NEW KNOWLEDGE:** Find a practitioner who is willing to listen and learn with you. If you present a new concept to the practitioner and he or she immediately shuts you down with no reason, that person might not be a lifelong learner! Is your practitioner willing to say, "I do not know about this [new concept you just presented], but I will look it up and let you know."

7) **ARE THEY WILLING TO REFER?:** This is a key factor in searching for natural medicine practitioners: Do they feel they have all the answers? Are they willing to refer you to another practitioner (including a Western medicine doctor)? If any practitioner believes that he or she has all the answers for your entire well-being, you will want to be cautious. As I mentioned above, do not put expectations upon your provider to have knowledge outside his or her scope. You would never expect a cardiologist to do brain surgery.

8) **WHAT DOES YOUR HEART SAY?:** I remember going into a practitioner's office in Iowa with a doctor friend to learn a specific new technique. As I met the new practitioner, he was wearing a giant pentagram necklace, and a quick glance around his office and its decorations indicated to me that I did not want

to be anywhere near this man! You could tell that he was heavily involved in the occult and other elements that I did not want to expose myself to. I quickly exited that office and never returned. The same discernment needs to follow you as you pursue alternative medicine practitioners.

9) **IS THEIR LIFE IN BALANCE?:** We say at our office all the time that life is about balance. EVERY aspect of a person's life needs to be in balance. If you walk into a practitioner's clinic and it ischaotic and unorganized, or if the practitioner is unkempt, rude, nasty, or negative, is that representing balance? Do people speak highly of that person in your community? Are the clinic's employees friendly? Are they treating you like a dollar sign or a person? Do you feel like they are listening to you and your concerns, and treating you specifically or just like the status quo?

10) **ASK LIKE-MINDED PEOPLE:** Though the Internet is a powerful resource, it is not automatically the first place to find out about the type of practitioner for whom you are looking. It might be the first place to search for a specific type of practitioner in your area, but do not necessarily trust everything you read. There are companies that practices can utilize to increase their rating on sites like Google, Yelp, and other online review portals. Read the reviews carefully to see what the people are really saying. Are they disgruntled because of a wait in the waiting room? Are they disgruntled because the services cost them money? Are they disgruntled because of something that was out of the control of the clinic? Are they happy because they received a free bottle of water, or are they happy because of the service, answers, and/ or hope they received? In a world of fast technology and even quicker entitlement, we are fast to critique and then believe much of what we read—true or not.

As you are searching for your next provider, ask your like-minded friends whom they would go to for (insert issue here).

Ask them why they would recommend that specific practitioner. Ask them what specific things the practitioner treated them for and the subsequent results.

11) **BUILD A TEAM:** Consider that your goal is to improve your health, whether that is to get well from an existing condition or to just maintain good health through a healthy lifestyle of proper care for your body given you by your Creator. You need to look at practitioners as the team that is helping you attain that goal. Drugs/therapies/supplements do not heal you. They may assist your body toward healing, but it is ultimately the response of your body to move toward that healing process. More than one type of therapy and/or practitioner may be needed to assist you in that process. Do not expect too much from any one person you have gone to for treatment. He or she may or may not be part of the team you are building for the healthy goal you have for yourself. As you visit a new practitioner or seek a new therapy, always ask, "Is this it?!"

12) **RECORD YOUR HEALTH HISTORY:** In order to give your practitioner as much valuable information about yourself as possible, it is important to write down your health history. As you think back on various ailments/conditions/reactions that you have had throughout your life, those memories may help you to begin to piece together related incidents. Your practitioner will then be able to connect some dots and assist in the overall healing of your body. Remember that this is a holistic approach to healing, so considering various triggers and stressors in your life is also helpful in putting together the most effective plan to move you toward optimal health.

Be aware that oftentimes when swimming against the stream as it relates to medicine, there are people, and even your close family, who will question your decisions. You own your health and ultimately you are responsible for it. You will be your greatest advocate for your own care. Know what you are doing and why you are doing it—not just because "Dr. So-and-So recommends it."

Choices in alternative medicine should not be an issue that would cause a family to break apart. Though I believe that everyone would benefit from treating the body holistically, I have many friends and some family members who do not share this same belief. This is not worth breaking fellowship over. You all should still be able to eat Thanksgiving dinner together without fighting about healthcare. The apostle Paul talked about "knowing in part." Knowledge is given and received by people at various speeds. Show others the same level of graciousness that you would expect extended to you!

Now that we have the basics out of the way, let us dig into some different types of practitioners and what they treat. A quick web search of "complementary and alternative medicine" (CAM) will yield a number of results.

TRADITIONAL CAM THERAPIES:

Acupuncture—The practice of acupuncture has been around for centuries. It was always revered as science until the late fourth century when Taoism took it over and added to the healing science involved. Mainstream Christianity for centuries has struggled with acupuncture as I did. But again, it was God who created healing and who so intricately designed the body.

According to the University of Miami Health System here is a list of common conditions treated with acupuncture:

Overall, the Chinese have mapped the presence of 361 acupoints in the major meridians. Below is a list of conditions and circumstances for which people commonly find acupuncture treatment to be effective.

General: Allergies, Asthma, Sinusitis, Headaches, TMJ, Back Pain, Sciatica, Musculoskeletal Problems, Insomnia, Anxiety, Dizziness, Depression, High Blood Pressure, Chronic Fatigue, Fibromyalgia, Addictions, Indigestion, Constipation, Sexual Dysfunction, Post-Operative Recovery, Palliative Care.

Women's Health: Menstrual Irregularities, Menopause, Conception Difficulties, Pregnancy, Childbirth, Lactation Difficulties, Postpartum, Ovarian and Uterine Problems.

Men's Health: Prostate, Infertility, Impotence.

Pediatrics: Asthma, Cough, Digestive Problems, Behavioral Problems, Ear Infections, Sleep Problems.

Preventative Health: Prevention, Stress Management, Wellness, Seasonal Attunement

Acupuncture is recognized by the National Institute of Health (NIH) and the World Health Organization (WHO) to be effective in the treatment of a wide variety of medical problems. Below is a list of disorders for which acupuncture is effective (according to the NIH):

Muscle, Bone and Nerve Pain and Diseases, Sprains / Strains, Back Pain, Leg Pain, Foot Pain, Stiff Shoulders and Neck, Lumbago, Sciatica, Tennis Elbow, Carpal Tunnel syndrome and Painful Joints, TMJ, Toothache, Headache and Migraines, Rheumatism, Arthritis Facial Paralysis, Bell's Palsy, Fibromyalgia

Obstetrics and Gynecology: Menstrual Pain and Cramping, PMS, Menopause, Infertility, Fetal Malposition

Addictions: Tobacco, Narcotics, Alcohol, Weight Loss

Diseases of the heart and blood vessels: Angina, High blood pressure, Obesity, Drug addiction, Smoking

Digestive disorders: Indigestion, Stomach ulcers, Gall stones, Diarrhea, Constipation, Nausea and vomiting, Irritable Bowel Syndrome

Diseases of the respiratory system: Allergies, Asthma, Bronchitis, Sinusitis

Diseases of the nervous system: Stroke, Neuralgia, Stress, anxiety, depression and other nervous disorders, Nerve paralysis, Headaches/migraines[186]

Though I have a few things I would add to this list, I think this list is fairly comprehensive.

Homeopathy—According to https://hpathy.com/abc-homeopathy/what-is-homeopathy-definition-and-details/:[187]

Homeopathy is a medical science developed by Dr. Samuel Hahnemann (1755–1843), a German physician. It is based on the principle that "like cures like." In simple words, it means that any substance, which can produce symptoms in a healthy person, can cure similar symptoms in a person who is sick. This idea is referred to as the "Law of Similars," and was understood by Aristotle and Hippocrates and mentioned in ancient Hindu manuscripts. It was Hahnemann, however, who turned it into a science of healing.

The World Health Organization estimates that homeopathy is used by 500 million people worldwide, making it the second most widely used medicine in the world.

In England, France, Germany and the Netherlands, homeopathy is included in the National Health Service.

In France, 18,000 physicians prescribe homeopathic remedies. There are seven medical schools offering post grad degrees in homeopathy and all 23,000 pharmacies carry homeopathic remedies.

In England, 42% of British physicians refer patients to homeopaths. The Royal family has used homeopathy for three generations. There are currently five homeopathic hospitals, and the oldest, the Royal London Homeopathic Hospital, has been there for 100 years.

India has over 70,000 board certified homeopathic physicians, hundreds of homeopathic hospitals and clinics and many homeopathic medical schools.

In Germany, 20% of Physicians prescribe homeopathic remedies.

In the Netherlands, 45% of physicians consider homeopathy effective.

Homeopathy is also practiced in Vienna, Scotland, New Zealand, Australia, Canada, Russia, Brazil, Argentina, Mexico, Pakistan, Greece, Belgium.

I agree with the list from https://hpathy.com/abc-homeopathy/ homeopathic-faq/ on "What ailments can be treated by Homeopathy?"[188]

Almost all ailments are amenable to homeopathic treatment. But Homeopathy is best known for its ability to treat chronic ailments. The reason for this is that Homeopathy is the only system of medicine which offers curative treatment (not palliative) in many chronic ailments which have been declared 'incurable' by other schools of medicine. Be it skin disease, chronic gastric and intestinal disorders, chronic fatigue syndrome, migraine, asthma, allergic disorders, menstrual complaints, other hormonal disorders, arthritis, psychological disorders etc. etc. All these and many more chronic ailments have been affected curatively by Homeopathy. The only major limiting factors are 1. Gross structural and pathological changes. 2. Very low vitality of the patient. 3. Unavoidable presence of certain causative or maintaining factors.

Then Homeopathy is also known to make surgery unnecessary on many occasions. Many tonsils, adenoids, appendices etc. have been saved with Homeopathy. Benign tumors and renal stones also respond well to homeopathic treatment.

Naturopathy—Uses natural remedies and non-invasive remedies to promote self-healing. A visit to a local health food store can probably get you a phone number of a local naturopath. Standardly, a naturopath has a doctoral-level degree.

Chinese or Oriental medicine—Though this is a broad category, there are many different Oriental medicine and Chinese practices and products that we use in our office. Traditional Chinese medicine (TCM for short) has been used in China for more than 2,500 years and includes a mix of herbal medicine, acupuncture, massage, exercise, and dietary therapy. It is based upon the body's vital energy as it circulates through various channels or meridians. (Some of these same energy points are used in massage, reflexology, and acupuncture.) Obviously, since this is the traditional method of medicine in China, a vast number of things have been and are treated through TCM.

BODY ALTERNATIVE MEDICINE:

Chiropractic and Osteopathic Medicine—Daniel David Palmer was the founder of chiropractic medicine in 1895 in Davenport, Iowa. It specifically treats the mechanical disorders and dislocations of the musculoskeletal system. There are many different styles of chiropractic, and even some different techniques that have been developed that have seen great results for many people. Obviously, I am a chiropractor and believe firmly in its effectiveness.

I have personally seen chiropractic help people with injuries, arthritis, asthma, neck pain, back pain, carpal tunnel syndrome, sinus issues, constipation, colic, ear infections, gastrointestinal dysfunction, headaches, herniated disc, hip pain, menstrual dysfunction, neurodevelopmental conditions, pinched nerves, reflux, sciatica, scoliosis, stress, and whiplash.

Massage—Just as chiropractic care treats the bones, massage treats the muscles. Since not all massage therapists are created equally, it is wise to seek out a massage therapist who can address your specific needs.

One method of massage that has been offered in our office is called myofascial release (MFR therapy), which treats skeletal muscle immobility and pain. Various methods of massage can help with relaxation, circulation, muscle tightness, aches, pains, flexibility, range of motion, energy, scar tissue release, and more.

Physical Therapy—Though not considered an alternative medicine or treatment, I would be remiss to exclude physical therapy. Oftentimes, a good physical therapist can help a person with gait, balance, joint pain, dizziness, strength issues, etc. Finding a quality physical therapist who will treat you with hands-on therapy might be part of your wellness journey.

Body Movement—Like other wellness therapies, various exercise programs have been labeled as bad voodoo throughout the years as well. Before becoming involved in a specific exercise program, consider your specific needs and abilities to keeping fit. Be cognizant of what you are getting involved in, but do not underestimate the power of moving your body and getting your circulation and flexibility going. Proper exercise is important, especially in our screen-based society in which we live! Go take a walk—at least get up and move. The more you move, the healthier you will be.

Reflexology—Reflexology is way more than a foot massage. It utilizes pressure to the feet, face, and hands to restore blood flow to the various meridians of the body, all which are present in the hands, feet, and face. Reflexology has been known to help with stress, blood pressure, pain, digestive issues, depression/anxiety, insomnia, hormonal issues, and more. If I were looking for a reflexologist, I would want to make sure he or she had some clinical training and not just for relaxation.

DIET AND HERBS:

Dietary supplements—As I mentioned in my story above, whole food natural supplements are crucial medicine for the body. We have some specific whole food supplements that we use at our office that we believe to be the best at what they do. Potentially there are others out there that can operate with the same or near the same efficacy. A large portion of our practice is based upon the proper use of dietary supplements. Actually, this is one of the powerplants to our practice. Speaking directly to each of these supplements would require volumes of books.

If you are planning on embarking on this journey to natural wellness, please understand this is a step that cannot be skipped. The importance of your provider understanding how the body can process organic (relating to or derived from living matter) vs. inorganic (minerals) substances and the difference between synthetically created (in a lab) vs. whole food (in the ground) supplements is paramount.

Herbal Medicine—Oftentimes herbs are used as a means to get your body and its energy flowing in the right direction. Think of them as a rapid-response team. Herbal medicine can get you over the hump that can then be carried forward with dietary supplements and other treatments.

Nutrition and Diet—Sometimes we underestimate the toxic effects of what we put into our bodies. Food allergies, food sensitivities, refined foods, "fortified with" synthetic vitamins and minerals, food additives, chemicals, and dyes are just some of the items we ingest on a regular basis not fully understanding the long-term effects that those items have on our bodies, our immune systems, our aches, our pains, and our well-being. IF YOU ARE NOT WILLING TO MAKE CHANGES IN THESE AREAS OF YOUR LIFE, YOU ARE POTENTIALLY WASTING YOUR TIME AND MONEY TOWARD BETTER HEALTH.

Do not expect this to be easy! I can almost guarantee you that if you want to reach optimum health, you will need to make some changes in your diet and consumption habits. It is on a weekly basis that I am encouraging people to make dietary changes in their lives and they leave my office in tears. They are crying because they are in bondage to the sugars, grains, and other fillers that in their mind are making them happy, but their bodies are telling a different story.

Aromatherapy—Essential oils were mankind's first medicine. The use of essential oils is found in ancient Egyptian hieroglyphics, Chinese manuscripts, and in biblical references. Essential oils are produced from plants and become the very "essence" of the plant, thus the name essential oils. Many essential oils have bacterial, viral, and germ-killing properties. Most can also stimulate the immune system response by increasing white blood cell production. Many people have found great relief from many ailments through aromatherapy.

Though there are a few direct-sales companies out there promoting their essential oils as the best, it is crucial to make sure that whatever essential oils you are using are properly extracted for the use that you intend for them. It is always wise to choose USDA organic oils. Some oils can be ingested or applied topically with a carrier oil. Diffusing is also beneficial. There are entire books in the libraries and bookstores that will give you the many uses and benefits of essential oils. Just like with anything, you need to make sure you know what you are doing, the effects of what you are using, and possible contraindications of the products you are using. You will also want to be careful that you are not using an essential oil fragrance that someone nearby would find unpleasant.

MIND THERAPY:

Biofeedback/Neurofeedback—Again, I know that this is a controversial category and one that you will have to research, get advice on, and determine if it is part of your health journey.

I will speak directly to neurofeedback for a minute. About two years ago, we brought this technology into our office and have seen amazing results with depression, anxiety, sleep issues, fear, dizziness, cloudy-thinking, traumatic-brain injuries, ADD/ADHD, concussions, focus, etc.

EMDR—Though at first glance, a passerby may improperly see EMDR to be hypnosis, it is certainly not that! EMDR stands for eye movement desensitization and reprocessing. It is a form of psychotherapy developed by Francine Shapiro in 1988 that uses bilateral stimulation to assist clients processing disturbing thoughts and beliefs. I have heard of many great outcomes from people who have faced emotional trauma in their lives and this trauma began a downward slope of physical issues as a result. EMDR was a very effective treatment of the mind, which allowed me to then further treat the body.

Counseling—Again, this is not considered to be a CAM therapy, but do not underestimate the value of good counsel. Needing to go to counseling is not admitting that you are weak. There are counselors specifically trained in various areas such as eating disorders, PTSD, and brain injuries, as well as emotional needs. Going to the right therapist can make you stronger and bring healing in your life faster.

Setting Yourself Up for Success

The road to health and a healthy lifestyle is a lifelong journey. There will be potholes in the road and sometimes entire bridges that are out. Do not think for a second that I believe that all Western medicine doctors are bad. They have their place in your journey, just like these alternative medicine providers do too. Thanks for letting me share with you my journey of "this isn't it" to "THIS IS IT"! I firmly believe that it was because of my bad reaction to the sulfa drugs that God molded me into the person that I am today. Because of that experience, I have been able to be used by God to see many people healed from their infirmities.

You are on the right track by seeking out knowledge and wisdom regarding your health! Remember: Healing is God's to begin with! He created your body to heal. This does not always happen at the speed in which we would prefer it, but there is Hope—Hope eternal, through Jesus Christ.

Dr. Matthew Sams, DC, FIACA

Branson, Missouri USA

About the Author: Dr. Matthew Sams (DC, FIACA) was born and raised in Chariton, Iowa. He graduated from Palmer College of Chiropractic in 1994. Following chiropractic college, he practiced in Ankeny, Iowa, for five years. In August of 1999, he decided that Branson, Missouri, was where his heart was. Dr. Sams specializes in many different techniques. He feels that what the patient needs varies from person to person. His techniques consist of Diversified, Gonstead, Thompson, Activator, Acupuncture, Nutrition, Kinesio Taping and teaching education and health through radio programs and classes. Dr. Sams has a passion for helping his patients get the best out of life.

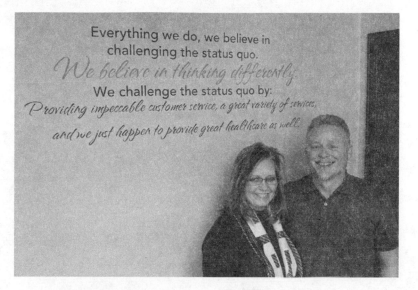

Dr. Matthew Sams and wife Tricia standing in front of the mission statement at their Healing Arts Center in Branson, Missouri. The statement reads: "Everything we do, we believe in challenging the status quo. We believe in thinking differently. We challenge the status quo by: Providing impeccable customer service, a great variety of services, and we just happen to provide great healthcare as well."

14

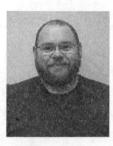

Dr. Joshua Vance
DC, MTAA

It was Sunday afternoon two summers ago and I was taking a short nap. I had been under a lot of stress due to meetings and commitments. I seldom ever take a nap because it usually makes me more tired and disrupts my normal cycle. My youngest daughter burst into the bedroom and said, "Daddy, there are fire trucks in the back pasture. Dazed, I said "What?" I thought she was playing a trick on me. We live out in a secluded area that has no homes or streets behind us. We have one close neighbor, but the rest are hundreds of yards away. It is completely foreign to us to have anyone on our property who is not invited. We are separated from our neighbors by tree lines on both sides. She was persistent and told me to get up and see. Half asleep, I rolled out of bed thinking I was being duped by my trickster. As I looked out the window, I noticed my back pasture was engulfed in flames. I threw my shoes on and rushed outside to see why that was happening. There were several rural fire trucks driving right behind my house into the burning flames. My heart was pounding as I rushed to the back area while feeling helpless. All I could do was pray that our house and barn would be unharmed and the fire department would be able to squelch the grass that was engulfed.

Have you ever been that close to an out-of-control fire? Maybe you have had firsthand experience seeing the destruction up close or seeing the destruction it has left behind. I was amazed at how quickly it spread with just a little wind and some dormant dry grass. We had been dry for a while and were desperately needing some rain. My neighbor had been doing a controlled burn on his property when the wind picked up and the dead grass suddenly took off. It was under control for a while and he has some knowledge of fire, being a volunteer on a rural fire department. Then suddenly there was no controlling the flames. They crossed the tree line and forged ahead with nothing but fuel in its path. He was smart enough to immediately call the fire department, as he saw how rapidly the flames jumped. I am grateful to the rural volunteer fire department for rushing out to help save our property and possibly our lives. They put out the flames using tanker trucks and were able to contain it before it could reach any of my neighbors' fields or dwellings.

I stood from my house watching the smoke rise from the charred pasture and thought what if we didn't know the field was on fire? What if it was at night and we were asleep? How would I put this out if I was alone? What if the volunteers were farther away and the fire had more time to burn? So many factors could have changed the outcome for the better or worse.

Here is the application. If the soil had been moist, then maybe the fire would have put itself out. If there was a way to reduce the fuel, such as less wind, then it would have stayed contained. If someone had been able to discuss and warn my neighbor about waiting for the right time or season, maybe then the soil could have been more fire resilient. The worst thing I could have done was run to my barn and grab all the gas cans I could get my hands on to attempt to put out the fire using more fuel or grab an extension cord and fan to blow it out. I know these seem ridiculous, but if people don't know any better, they could have furthered the destruction even though they thought it was helping. This is the current scenario we find ourselves in.

Being a physician in the current healthcare arena, I have had a front-row seat to view the health status of my community. I do not make a claim that all people are grouped into one category, but I do pay attention to trends. Witnessing my parents passing at an early age allowed me to have retrospection into the current predicament we all are facing.

Some Observations

Most of the decline I have seen and statistics I have read over the years tie back to a specific trend. There was a tipping point that seems to alter the physical, mental, and/or emotional stability of the now ill. Medical professionals state that majority of the diagnosis comes from the history. I hear people say that it is because of their age (such as "I am 40 or 50 now"). There are remarkable cases of people who seem to do better than others during this transition, and I often wondered why? Also, why does it seem that we are seeing children with illnesses such as hypertension and type II diabetes that we often see in middle age or even in the elderly? Do certain factors make us age faster? Are we genetically weaker than our ancestors? If so, why? Is the environment in which we find ourselves now more toxic than it was a century ago? Let's consider some thoughts about life today.

Food

We have two dogs and two cats that live indoors with us. My daughters are animal lovers. They love almost every wild creature that God has created, and I love my daughters. We have an indoor litter box. The two dogs constantly stick their heads into the cats' litter box and retrieve a small morsel, then run and lay down on the landing at the stairs to enjoy their little treasure. I never thought that as a grown man I would constantly have to say the words "stop eating cat turds." No matter where we place the litter box, the dogs are drawn to eat from it. I know this is dramatic, but dogs can't live on cat turds alone.

Do we get the same nutrition from our food that our great-grandparents consumed? With the advancement of research and technology in farming practices, farmers have become much better at drought resistance and stopping/slowing destruction by plant disease. I respect the reason it is done: to maximize the yield of the crop, which aids in making it profitable. Many of the farmers I talk with discuss how difficult it is to stay profitable in today's farming environment. But does the research on food production look more at yield production or quality of nutrition to consumers? If you were purchasing vitamins and had a report on the total availably of nutrients and cost analysis, would you choose a lesser brand that would give you 40 percent of the nutrition because it is cheaper? Would you solely depend on price? Maybe you would make your selection based on how it looks, or what it tastes like. What about who made it and how it was processed?

Not all things are as they appear. We can make beautiful floral arrangements that, with the unaided eye, appear real. A bumble bee will know the difference. We have all purchased something and later realized that the package was very well done—so well done, in fact, that it made us make a decision without ever handling the product. What about people? Some people may look like they are healthy, fit, and even kind or compassionate, and later we realize that we have misjudged them or their circumstance.

Food is no different. If we do not grow or produce our own food, we are just accepting that all things are standard. Is this the same assumption we should make about people? What about cars, tools, or jewelry? There are different qualities of jewelry, and we often will pay more for purer metal or clarity. It has much to do with the purity or density (nutrition).

There are brilliant people whose job it is to make food taste better because we as the consumer will not buy their products because they are not palatable. Research is even done on specifics of color. If we won't buy the product, those people will not continue to have a position. If you are raising cattle for your own consumption, would you give it the best food? What if you were going to just sell the cattle? Would you spend extra to make sure the nutrition is in your livestock? No one will care more about what is in your food than you will, and not all food is equal.

Shopping at your local grocery store will also confirm that not all food is created equal. We pay more for better grades of beef and to buy truly organic vegetables. I believe our system has been developed and driven by what we consume and because of our buying habits. We show up, and this is already in motion. If we do not purchase certain products, the companies that sell it will not continue to manufacture these items because of simple supply and demand. It may be great for you, but no one buys it, then there really would be no need to produce it. I know there are other factors we as the consumer look at when selecting any product. Price, package, taste, and even emotion all play into our decision of selection. Food is no different in our process, but much of it comes down to taste.

Think in terms of a business. Would you set up your business process based on what would be the hardest to sell and give a return on your investment? Would you pay attention to trends and lean the direction as to make the most of your energy? Take fishing, for example. Nobody likes preparing and spending time to catch fish and walk away with no action. We tend to go where the action is and use the "bait" that will bring about the action on the end of our rod. That is why I believe in order to eat better quality of food, it will cost us more money. Our current scenario of food manufacturing is set up to produce a high yield so that most consumers will buy their products. Buying truly organic may cost more, because the trend has not completely tipped that direction yet. Naively, I hope someday that trend will be in favor of more nutritious and truly organic food. Until then, I must do my research for my family and make better nutritional choices, possibly spend more at the local grocery store, and grow/raise my own food.

A simple food observation: The foods that are rich in carbohydrates seem to be the least expensive. Shopping with larger amounts of meat in your cart will lead to a higher bill at the register. If the majority of our decision is based on cost and taste, we will most likely have a basket full of foods that are less nutritious. We are often shortsighted in our thinking. Consider this statement: Most chronic degenerative disease is directly linked to lifestyle. Chronic degenerative conditions like obesity, diabetes (type II), hypertension, and cardiovascular disease are just a few. Lifestyle is the summation of our choices up to this point of our life. Food choices, stress, daily exercise, and career choice make up our lifestyle. We learn what is an acceptable lifestyle from our family as we develop. This is where I connected the dots for myself. I read an article several months ago stating that cardiovascular disease starts in the second decade of life. So, as I pondered my second decade, I was in college eating foods rich in carbohydrates because of cost containment, pushing my physical and mental abilities because I thought my body could handle the stress, and choosing to exercise less because of time—all this may have started a smoldering fire.

Let's say that in our teenage years we started to develop some bad habits. We love to eat pancakes with syrup, cereal for breakfast, drink a two-liter of soda a day, avoid vegetables because we don't like the taste, can't afford to eat meat, play video games for hours on end, and the only exercise we get is walking to and from our vehicle with a little physical education class at school a few days a week. Maybe we stay up all night on the weekends binge-watching our favorite TV shows while eating some comfort foods or gaming into the late hours. Later that decade, our stress levels go up due to the burden or demands our job or schooling put on us. We become more dependent upon technology daily, so we use it for both our job and our recreational time on social media. If we care about our physical appearance, we may join a fitness club to help, but that is a small contribution to our overall health. That sounds a lot like my college years, and that's where the fire began. We start to become ill and tired, and we run around kind of in a fog and don't make the greatest choices. Could even our lifestyle and diet lead down a path to moral decay and poor choices just because of the above scenario? Maybe we have "stinking thinking" because of the smoke in our eyes from the fire of our lifestyle. Just a thought.

Let's call it like we see it. We use terms like "chocoholic," carb-o-holic, and sweet tooth. Comfort foods are always rich in carbs and fats. When was the last time you were stressed out and thought "that's it, I'm done; give me the vegetables"? Carbohydrates(sugars) cause a spike in insulin, which is a powerful hormone. I remember when my father was diagnosed with type II diabetes. He would sneak candy and even lie about it. This was not a normal practice for him given his rich Christian belief. While in chiropractic school, I remember a teacher stating that diabetics will lie about their diet because they can't control their sugar cravings. Much of my time evaluating patients' blood labs is spent on blood-sugar dysregulation. I see overwhelming clinical evidence that many of our health-related issues trend because of an unhealthy relationship with sugar. Honestly, most celebrations in our family involve food, and the majority comes in the form of carbohydrates. What about yours?

Environment

Do we live in a more toxic society? We live in a fast-paced life compared to fifty or one hundred years ago. We go in early and leave late, and still have families to feed. We want our food sooner rather than later and depend on convenience more than quality. This is not an attempt to make you feel guilty; it is the cultural position we find ourselves in. Do simple things like vine-ripened tomatoes from your garden have more nutrition? Does packaging matter? What about how we heat and prepare our food? Does the soil have less nutrition or more contaminants? It is difficult to make some of these comparisons because certain technology wasn't available a century ago. What about the effects on our bodies from sitting behind a desk eight hours a day and the use of electronics that make our life more productive? Many sites on the web state that "sitting is the new smoking." Could the dependence on our bottom position be putting our health in the bottom position? I administer treatment to younger children due to GPS issues—"gaming posture syndrome" (this is what I call it). Kids sit in front of a gaming console for hours on end and that leads to spinal problems and has an effect on their overall health. People today have "tech neck" or "text neck" due to the long hours spent in front of an electronic device. How about time spent on social media? Not mentioning the effects on our mental well-being of constantly being "plugged in" to potentially negative mental or emotional stimuli. I have a dear friend who is involved in an electronic software company; he has watched his health decline because of his high-stress environment, constant seated position, and declining job satisfaction. What about basic human interaction? How long has it been since you have had a conversation with another human without distractions such as a phone or Internet? Maybe you live in an urban setting with "noise pollution" or "urban convergence."

My wife and I travel to sneak away at times from our busy life, and we love northern Arkansas. It is a short distance for us and we have been there many times. We went on a guided tour at the Crescent Hotel in Eureka Springs, a hotel and area that are rich in history. On the tour, the guide discussed the many "healing" springs in the town, and said that wealthy people from all over the country would descend upon the area when they were sick because of the waters' restorative health properties. The guide made a remarkable statement that getting away to the secluded countryside and eating the local produce probably had more to do with their recovery than the springs themselves.

I have family members who reside in the Denver, Colorado, area and love to come to our home in southern Missouri. For this reason, they hope to someday move here because of the relaxing time it offers as an alternative to their normal "on-the-go" lifestyle. Could this be a major contribution to their health?

I tell my kids that you can glean much information about a future spouse by considering the soil they were grown in—what type of family life they had and what their early relationships were like. We've all been shaped by our experiences and the ups and downs of life. That is what makes someone "seasoned." Kids watch their parents for an example of how to engage with the world and how to have relationships. The cliché, "an apple doesn't fall far from the tree," is something I use many times in trying to evaluate standards. A good tree produces good fruit. I'm also aware that some of my mannerisms and habits are accepted by my children as normal or proper. This can have a huge impact on their choices about health, environment, career, and habits. I have had to make different choices for my environment because I did not want my parents' health issues or their chronic illness.

Stress

The word "stress" immediately brings to mind things like money, deadlines, or arguments. All of these areas can be stressors that we rename in many ways. Grief, sickness, worry, and saving face (pride) with others' opinions are other factors that increase our levels of stress. What about negative thoughts and emotions such as depression, anxiety, and fear? It takes very little time to read a news article or watch a television program that then starts the cycle of "what if?". There are good responses to stress and detrimental ones that lead to negative effects on our bodies. When a certain type of life event comes, we have been equipped to elevate our physical body to meet the level of stress and then return to our baseline. When the event continues for days, weeks, months, or even years, then there can be a toll on our physical and emotional/mental wel-lbeing.

Stress increases specific hormones in our body such as epinephrine/norepinephrine to meet its needs. When we're stressed, our blood-sugar levels start to rise, as does our cholesterol in response to the stress-inducing outside or inside stimulus. Our heart rate may also elevate and our blood pressure may increase—and this is all a natural reaction to an abnormal stimulus. The body is constantly trying to react to the stimulus set before it and maintain balance. The term for this is "homeostasis." When we think we are being chased by a lion, we want these body functions to be occurring so we may escape the danger we perceive. We only have a limited amount in storage, and when we are chronically "running" from our danger, we need to recover. Our bodies learn to be proficient at maintaining the balance until it runs out of the ability to handle the stress and no longer can maintain homeostasis.

The inability to handle the load prompts a person to reach out in desperation for help. This is the time a person often needs help, someone who can look n from the outside and evaluate why the body cannot withstand even simple tasks of life or activities without drastic recovery methods. Finding a doctor is usually the next step.

In any given day, all of us deal with certain stimuli that trigger our stress system. We can narrowly miss another car on the road, hear of a loved one in crisis, face a deadline requiring us to work harder and faster than anticipated, have a longstanding sickness place a burden on our physical body, or maybe all four. When your body elevates to meet that need, but fails to return to your normal resting state, there is a problem. The long duration of being under that load leads to the body coping with the increased physiological response.

Our bodies secrete hormones to react to the stimulus. One such hormone is cortisol, which is made in the adrenal gland atop the kidneys and controlled through the brain and under nervous-system control. When we're sick or under stress, cortisol is secreted. Cortisol is the body's natural "anti-stress" and "anti-inflammation" response. Remember, the body is always trying to maintain homeostasis. When we experience stress, this is the way our body returns to the normal level and "heals" from the stimuli. When cortisol is elevated for long periods, it dramatically affects all the systems of the body. It increases blood-sugar levels linking to elevated heart rate and blood pressure, impairs wound healing by the immune system, upsets electrolyte balance, increases gastric acid secretion, and disrupts sleep patterns as well as mood. Long-standing elevation leads to muscle wasting due to its effect on amino acid uptake by muscles and reducing bone formation. I encourage the reader to look up the known effects of elevated cortisol on the human body.

Factors that increase the production of cortisol are infections, caffeine, poor sleep, prolonged repetitive physical strain of the body(inflammation), trauma, mental stress, obesity, and consumption of alcohol. So let's paint a picture together. A person has a job that brings him little satisfaction and requires him to achieve high expectations. Maybe his job requires standing or sitting all day. His home life includes the constant struggles associated with raising children, family stress, and credit-card debt, which prompts him to pick up another shift or second job to ease the financial burden. He can't afford to quit his job or take a vacation. He is constantly running to provide for his family by grocery shopping, taking the kids to practice, dealing with unresolved feelings of the fight he had with his loved one last night. While shopping, he fills the cart with foods that taste good but are not nutritious and are pro-inflammatory in nature. He picks up foods that elevate sugar level as comfort foods and a bottle of wine or six-pack of beer to drown the stress for the evening. He has been sitting behind a desk eating chips for a snack because he becomes irritable when he gets hungry. He doesn't have time to exercise, and because of the long hours behind the desk and taking care of the family needs, he doesn't have thirty minutes a day to go to the gym—or he can't afford the expense. Then, he gets the cold or flu doesn't have the time or money to be sick. Healing does not come quickly and he wonders why he doesn't recover quickly, like he used to. He is laid up in bed with the worries of how he will get it all done or pay the bills. He starts to feel tired and run down all the time. When it comes to bedtime, maybe he can get to sleep, but he doesn't sleep all night. Later, he can't seem to go to sleep even though he feels exhausted. Morning coffee is now a staple, and the rule of the home is that no talks to him until he has had a cup of black sunshine. It seems as if he is always in a mental fog and doesn't know why he doesn't feel good. Eating and caffeine minimize the fog, but only temporarily. Or, say this person is a female. Her cycles become abnormal and her physical desire for her mate decreases. Her relationship with her husband now seems like a boxing match with pauses only between rounds. Because of the lack of physical exercise and being seated behind a computer, she starts gaining unwanted weight. She doesn't want to be intimate looking like this. She finds herself crying at every heart-tugging commercial or Hallmark card.. Her clothes don't fit anymore, and that is its own stressor. She finds herself being short with the people she loves, and all she wants to do is retreat to watch TV or play a game on her phone. Embarrassed by the way she may look, she fears and avoids social engagements. She starts to feel depressed because life is not the way she had planned. Nearly having an accident on the way to work leads her to want to crawl into bed until it is safe to come out. She gets on the computer and consults Dr. Google, and now the anxiety really kicks in. *What if I have this disease and it will affect my ability to sustain life as I know it?* she asks. She starts a

New Year's resolution to exercise, but it now hurts too much because of the inflammation. The guilt of not meeting the exercise quota now sets in and furthers the cycle. She doesn't have to eat much to gain weight, and it seems like even just smelling food now adds to the bulge. She is constantly on the edge of breakdown and develops a survival mentality. Hope is merely a dream that is interrupted by the reality of life. She becomes become negative or cynical towards life and those around her. If she gets a vacation, all she wants to do is hibernate in bed with an occasional food outing. Later on, cleaning the house is physically exhausting and adds more to the depressive cycle. She wishes she could retreat to a secret spot where no one could find her.

People suffering from stress like this often then make an appointment with a doctor to find out what is wrong—but nothing shows up on the tests. The doctor may state the stressed-out person should take an antidepressant for depression or anxiety. It helps maybe for a little while to normalize, but continues, requiring adjustment of the dosage. Maybe a second medication would work, but it merely maintains these feelings from going farther downhill for a time.

Any of this sound familiar?

Have you ever felt anguish over friends or loved ones who, if they would take some good advice and some initiative, could see improvement in their circumstances? When people are in the midst of the trials of life, they don't always think clearly or make good decisions. Often they retreat to a safe place that brings them comfort. I have always wondered why we do certain things (destructive habits) or eat certain foods (comfort foods) that only seem to worsen the long-term objective to recovery. Depending on our state of health, we can even recover from our bad choices. Sometimes these continue to worsen the already-wearied body and soul. Some people seem genetically able to endure more and some have better approaches to managing stress through healthy or more productive approaches.

How many times have you spilled your troubles to a trusted friend to get great advice that helps you make better decisions? In my opinion, that is what a doctor visit should resemble. Sometimes you are frantic and completely lost and need someone to lead you through a situation. Some people just need some good advice to help them get even better results.

Application

So what do we do? First, look at your current circumstances you find yourself. Look at a week of your life and your family's habits. Don't feel guilty because nobody knew to teach you how to care for your health. Are there things that can be improved? Are you so sick that you don't know where to start? Some of my patients are so unhealthy that just starting a workout would crash the system. Find good resources to learn about what you should put in your body. Get evaluated to see where you stand in your health. One patient stated the most devastating blow to an opinion is a number. We test so we will know otherwise; everything else is a guess. If you called me on the phone and told me you were lost in the woods, the first thing I would have to do is find you the map to give direction. Just imagine your navigation system telling you by using random directions. There must be a reference point, and often the "trees" occlude our view to a familiar path. That is why we need an "eye in the sky" to get us to our destination.

Finding an Advisor

Some people require medication and intensive approaches to begin healing or the path to recovery. When you finds yourself in a deep, dark hole, the first and foremosts step is to stop digging. You must accept your part in this path. If a person is drowning in water, unless he realizes he needs help or to make a change, a "life preserver" may be a nuisance or obstacle.

Some may be able to navigate it on their own while others may need an outside observer who has either walked this path or been down it with others.

Andy Stanley, senior pastor of Grace Baptist Church in Asheville, North Carolina, has said: "You are unique but your circumstances are not." Every person is different, and not all approaches work the same. I equate this to having many different roads to my destination. There are faster and slower routes that will take me to the same place. We often as observers try to figure out our path by a minute-to-minute assessment of our journey. Wouldn't it be a better approach to have someone with a guide? That is where a physician or trusted advocate comes in.

That's Not Normal

Many people may have sought advice from a healthcare professional due to their symptoms. They just don't feel right. After examination and lab evaluation, they leave their encounter disappointed because they are sick, but not sick enough to find it through a lab. Ranges are used specifically on lab values to spot outliers. During your body's wonderful attempt to maintain homeostasis, if it cannot do so, then we see values creeping out of bounds. Out of clinical range, usually listed as "H" for "high" or "L" for "low," means "sick" and "dying, and in a hurry." Sick means not feeling well and symptomatic. Dying means the body cannot revert to normal (Hurry—need to do something quick!) Most traditional approaches to someone who is dying include medication and hospitalization. Realistically, that may be necessary to stop the decline of the condition, but it will not restore to complete health. Bodies that are healthy don't need medications, they need nutrition and a healthy lifestyle. Using a hospital as the only intervention for our health is like taking your car to the mechanic when it breaks down, but never checking the oil or doing routine maintenance until it won't drive and needs a wrecker to get it to the shop. Gas it up and drive into the ground.

I have heard of patients being told that they're not sick enough yet to treat. That doesn't make sense to me. Many people may find themselves saying they don't feel good, but the doctor says nothing is wrong. I don't believe we have an epidemic of malingerers. You will be the first to not feel right, but that, too, may be a later stage of a problem. Symptoms usually show up later than sooner.

We are looking at trends. It is like your kid in the front yard getting closer to the busy street. He may still be in the yard, but he's getting awfully close to that dangerous road.

When I am looking at blood labs, I am trying to find out why we are trending in a direction. On every target there is bull's-eye. We may be able to hit the target, but we are looking at the center. I use clinical range and optimum range. Outside of clinical range means your kid is in the road. Optimal range is where your body is at homeostasis. The closer I can make it to optimum means the more accurate my approach is—which is why I use routine labs on individuals to keep score for them. I expect that if I am using the correct approach, then lab values should be changing and having an impact on symptoms.

A Better Approach

The thought of taking a medication for the rest of my life just does not sit well with me. I am not against the use of medication when it is necessary. What I want from my doctor is to help restore my health so I will not need to be dependent upon an outside chemical. Some people may feel they will just take a specific drug the rest of their life and change nothing about their lifestyle. We may be able to patch the system for a season, but eventually the patch fails and requires a larger, more drastic approach. Type II diabetes is a classic example of management more than correction. Diabetes is a blood-sugar-regulation issue that can last for years. It is a major contributor to blindness, amputation, vascular disease, and early death. Patients don't usually die directly from diabetes, they die from the effects of diabetes. I discuss with patients that if you are a diabetic and continue to be a diabetic, it will shorten your estimated life expectancy by one-third. Many are coming to accept that many cases of type II diabetes can be reversible. How do they do it? Lifestyle. In our office, we are trying to catch the trend before patients become diabetic. The sooner we "cast weapons" for the war for their health, the easier it is to return to the baseline.

Let's not wait until the child reaches the street to do something about his safety. Be proactive in your approach. First, take some good advice about food choices, environment, and lifestyle. It is not your doctor's responsibility to stand over you at the grocery store or hold the stopwatch while you're running the track. We all must have an aspect of personal accountability. Find someone to hold you accountable.

Find a doctor who understands the difference between clinical range and optimum range. Clinical range can be the gray area for most. "I don't feel good, but my doctor says nothing is wrong" is something I hear regularly. The road to recovery many times will take time and run in the opposite direction, which is often up hill. It will require thinking differently and making other choices when it comes to your approach. The "pill for each ill" is not the approach that I think makes sense.

The sicker an individual, the more drastic the approach. The longer the illness has been in motion, the longer it will be to balance again. We can use therapeutic approaches to stop and turn the trend of our health. My goal is not to trade medications only for vitamins and supplements. The goal is to get better health through proper lifestyle. Often people use supplements only to not have to use medications, which can be good; but unless the lifestyle is changed, we are still only maintaining the lower level of health. There is no quicker way to feeling like we should than changing our lifestyle. Let's face it, it is so much easier to give a compound and send the patient home than to educate them why and what to do.

Stop fueling the fire. Call the fire department and get some help. Just think how ridiculous it would be for you, while the fire department is waging war against the flames that are engulfing your personal possessions, to go to the gas station and get all the gasoline you can bring to help put out the fire.

Much of the discussion in our office is how to use natural approaches to help patients regain their health and well-being. I never would recommend stop using a medication prescribed by another practitioner. What I am in pursuit of is to make help make patients' health good enough that they don't have to depend on medication.

The Titration Event

In chemistry class, I remember adding two clear liquid compounds into the same glass slowly over time, waiting for a color change. One clear liquid in a glass beaker with a single drop of a clear compound at a time—the goal was to see how much of one compound added at the rate of a single drop it would take before the compound changed to a different color. Drop, drop, drop, and then *boom!* The reaction happened and the liquid in the beaker was now blue. This maybe similar to our recovery: one drop at a time. We are looking for how to speed the reaction. This is what a change in lifestyle will look like.

The Great Physician and His Advisor

I think I can paint a clinical picture of why a believer can and should live a long and healthy life because of what it may do to cortisol levels.

People carry the guilt of past mistakes or of current struggles. They feel hopeless, unwanted, disconnected, and rejected. Maybe they are carrying a life of hurts or assaults by other terrible circumstances. They wonder, "Is this all there is to life?" The question "Am I cursed?" enters their mind. They have unresolved forgiveness in their heart or believe they have done something so horrible that there is no redemption. They believe there is no existence after death, and this is it. As they see their life coming closer to an end, they see their life achievements fading like the leaves on the tree as Fall appears. Maybe they are so desperate they cry out in the weakness because the burden is so heavy. They wish it was day because the nights are so lonely. They wish it was night because the burden of the day is overwhelming. Nothing goes right, and they have no peace or safety. At the end of their path, they cry out "God save me."

And there will be signs in the sun, in the moon, and in the stars; and on the earth distress of nations, with perplexity, the sea and the waves roaring; men's hearts failing them from fear and the expectation of those things which are coming on the earth, for the powers of the heavens will be shaken. (Luke 21:25–26)

Inasmuch then as the children have partaken of flesh and blood, He Himself likewise shared in the same, that through death He might destroy him who had the power of death, that is, the devil, and release those who through **fear of death were all their lifetime subject to bondage.** (Hebrews 2:14–15, emphasis added)

But know this, that in the last days perilous times will come: For men will be lovers of themselves, lovers of money, boasters, proud, blasphemers, disobedient to parents, unthankful, unholy, unloving, unforgiving, slanderers, without self-control, brutal, despisers of good, traitors, headstrong, haughty, lovers of pleasure rather than lovers of God, having a form of godliness but denying its power. And from such people turn away!For of this sort are those who creep into households and make captives of gullible women loaded down with sins, led away by various lusts, always learning and never able to come to the knowledge of the truth. (2 Timothy 3:1–7)

In the morning you shall say, "Oh, that it were evening!" And at evening you shall say, "Oh, that it were morning!" because of the **fear which terrifies your heart**, and because of the sight which your eyes see. (Deuteronomy 28:67, emphasis added)

Just take a journey reading through Deuteronomy 28 starting in verse 16 to the end. It paints a terrible picture of anxiety, disease, depression, and despair. Inflammation, fever, bodily pains, and mental anguish are individualized. This is not God's desire for us. Looking at all these things, I see the continuous inflammation and the sufferer's body trying to maintain homeostasis with cortisol, and it cannot produce enough.

Then one day, they had heard about this Savior from a friend who, remarkably, seems to be able to go through difficult life events and seems to have strength. She had a "past," but now is open and even regretful about it—not from a sense guilt, but from an overcoming confidence that it will not define her life. She constantly talks about her "new life" and how all the guilt she carried for many years has faded like stains on clothes after many washings. She leads a group at church and loves to talk about her testimony of how forgiven she is and the love that God has for her. She has an overwhelming confidence that God will bring her through the difficulties of this world, and she trusts in Him. She has a personal, loving relationship with the One who saved her, and she constantly looks at the day as to what He will bring. She has settled in her mind the aspect of eternity and believes deeply that this world is not her home. She believes her home to be beyond all she could dare ask or think, and the Lover of her soul is always with her. She always believes that all things will work out for her, because "He cares for her." She loves to sing and dance to songs about her great God and the Lover of her soul. She lights up with anticipation when she talks about where she will live eternally with the King. She no longer has a rejected mindset because God has given value to her life, and she tells Him how thankful she is by telling others of His glorious work. She even talks with Him anytime she wants, and He answers her prayers. Often, she admits they are answered better than she even asked. She has a peace about her, even when most think she should be worried. She spends time just sitting and thanking her Savior for all He has done. It is like she gains strength from doing so. Many people who knew her before say she is completely different person. She spends her time tending to her family and loves to help the less fortunate. Even when negative comments are said about her, she cares little, smiles knowingly, and states, "He cares for me." She is a rock, and prays earnestly for those around her that their "eyes" would be open. She doesn't worry about things like her coworkers and peers do. You can tell that she truly cares for people and rarely has anything negative to say. She is a giver of both her talents and resources, and people are constantly drawn to her. When she walks into the room, it lights up. She's always content, whatever circumstances she finds herself in.

> **Peace** I leave with you, My **peace** I give to you; not as the world gives do I give to you. **Let not your heart be troubled, neither let it be afraid**. (John 14:27, emphasis added)

> **Be anxious for nothing,** but in everything by **prayer** and supplication, **with thanksgiving,** let your requests be made known to God. (Philippians 4:6, emphasis added)

He sent His **word** and **healed** them, And delivered *them* from their destructions. (Psalm 107:20, emphasis added)

It is vain for you to rise up early, To sit up late, To eat the bread of sorrows; For so **He gives His beloved sleep**. (Psalm 127:2, emphasis added)

What lowers cortisol (stress, inflammation, chronic deg disease)? Music therapy, laughing, and dancing, to name a few. I would also venture to say some other areas, such as Scripture reading, praise, singing, worship (music/dancing), thanksgiving, security for eternal life, sense of community among a local church, acts of service, forgiving and being forgiven, extension of love such as hugs (physical contact), trusting in a Savior, rest (Sabbath). What about prayer, friendship, and fasting? I believe God has given these aspects from His Word for our benefit the most.

Thanksgiving—in all things give thanks (it may lower your cortisol and inflammation).

There is no question in my mind that being grateful is part of a long and healthy life. I remember giving a talk to a group of doctors around the Thanksgiving season. I had discussed the positive effects with chronic pain, depression, and anxiety by using a gratitude journal. I had found it very interesting that some researchers stated you could change the trajectory of your thought pattern and emotional behavior just with a simply ten-minute journal entry listing what you were grateful for on that day. I have used this as an adjunct in treatment to help people "hijack" their behavior or thought pattern. I am reminded always to "give thanks" in the New Testament, because this IS the will of God for you. I don't believe that God in any way feels inferior so that we must give Him thanks to puff Him up by human standards. I believe there is a benefit to us for giving thanks. When our heart is grateful to the overwhelming fact that Jesus purchased our freedom by suffering for us, it has a drastic effect on our body and mind. God is a giving Father who wants His children to be healthy and strong against the cares of this world. He is "joy," and we are to delight ourselves in Him. We are to enter into His presence with thanksgiving and praise (Psalm 100:4) Truly, I believe God has wired us to be grateful to Him for our benefit. Give it a try sometime and write down on paper for ten minutes what you are grateful for to your Heavenly Father and see how you feel for thirty days. A thanksgiving journal has immensely helped me keep calm during some of my most stressful times, and I have noted having a shorter fuse and easily being frustrated when I forgot it for a season. It takes me a few days to build up the benefit, but then I just feel at peace. Combined with Scripture reading, you may just have a powerful foundation for keeping your emotional stability and cortisol level lower.

Conclusion

I love the passage at the end of Psalm 91, which states, "Long life will I satisfy him and show him my salvation." Without the trust in a Savior for the redeeming of our mistakes and the belief of God for us and with us, there is no peace that surpasses all understanding that quiets our hearts and minds. Everything else is rearranging the deck chairs on the Titanic while the music plays.

This is more a marathon than a sprint, so start small. Evaluate your current position. What would you change about your lifestyle? Look at the trends you are setting for you and your family. Consider educating yourself on food. Apply some simple and easy steps to reverse the trend. Take some of the thoughts from above and start a new trend. Put the fires out. Get some help from people that have the understanding and training that can assist you in recovery.

I pray that your eyes are opened and that you may feel motivated to look differently into your future and health. May you truly have the peace that surpasses all understanding, and may it help with giving you and your family a strong foundation that will help them have a full and healthy life.

Dr. Joshua Vance CBP, MTAA

About the Author: Dr. Joshua W. Vance (DC, MTAA) is a chiropractic specialist in Republic, Missouri. He graduated with honors from Cleveland Chiropractic College, Kansas City in 1999. Having more than nineteen years of diverse experiences, especially in chiropractic, Dr. Vance affiliates with no hospital, and cooperates with other doctors and specialists in the medical group, Vance Chiropractic, Inc.

15

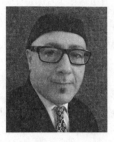

Dr. Ralph A. Umbriaco
DC, MsTOM, CNHP

If you had a choice between a pain-free, disease-free, happy, healthy, and productive life versus a life full of heaviness, sadness, misery, restricted movement, pain, anxiety, helplessness, hopelessness, fatigue and depression, which would you choose? Winston Churchill once said that, "The wealth of any nation can be measured by the health of her people." Interesting...let that sink in: The connection between being healthy and having the ability to leverage that health into something more fruitful... a valued and productive life. History has proven that, for the most part, everyone...sooner or later, has to die; however, where is it written or why do so many expect or believe that everyone has to die sick? Is "sickness" something that all of us are destined or required to experience? Is it unreasonable to consider or expect the possibility that health can, and perhaps maybe even "should" be, a natural, normal part of every-day life? Well, the answer to both of the above questions is both "yes" and "no." The outcome is conditional, based on your ability to choose and execute on either principles of disease and death or health and life. If you choose to be sick, f fine. It is not that difficult to do, as long as you meet certain requirements and criteria for disease to occur, then, given enough time, you will become successful at creating a diseased state or potential, and sickness will most likely occur. Happily, the con-verse is also quite true. If you wish to become or remain healthy, well, that is equally fine. It is really not that difficult to do, as long as you meet certain requirements and criteria for health to occur, then, given enough time, you will become successful at creating a healthier state or potential for well-being and health will also most likely occur. In the end, the choice is overwhelmingly ours: We can be sick or we can be healthy. It is our choice and our responsibility. The most deciding factor in determining our health future is our ability to recognize and choose life over death…health over disease. Which begs the question: "How, exactly, does one go about 'creating' life and health in a sick or diseased body or mind? By way of illustration, this concept can be viewed and examined as an equation that can look something like this: wisdom, understanding, and knowledge + personal responsibility and steward-ship = God-given health. If taken seriously and applied appropriately, the success of your efforts is almost a certain guarantee of incredibly improved health and wellness. If ignored or shunned, well, let's put it this way: As a "free-will agent," you have the right to jump out of an airplane without a parachute IF you so desire; however, once that choice is made, we do not always have to ability, luxury or the right to escape the negative consequences. Again, the choice is ours. The good news is we are all free-will agents with the ability to learn and choose, serv-ing a loving and Almighty God, under the blood sacrifice and with the power and instruction of the Holy Spirit. And under the capacities and potential of all of that, we can boldly proclaim and move forward in confidence to initiate personal emotional and lifestyle changes that can benefit us for the good, better, and best potentials that each of us possess. Benjamin Franklin is quoted as having once said, "God heals and the doctor bills." I believe this to be a true statement, especially after twenty-five years in practice. Yes, each practitioner has gone through years of rigorous training and competency exams. Yes, each practitioner can assist and educate the client and his or her body in the hopes of stimulating "the doctor within" to rise up and fulfill the call for repair of imbalanced systems. However, at the cellular level, it is the power of God and His intelligent design that we find most amazing and the true source of our healing and repair...and in that is much hope. So, does that mean that we are to sit by idly and wait patiently on the sidelines, hoping for God to notice us in our distress and expect that He should have compassion for us and fix us instantly with little or no effort on our part? Well, oddly enough, yes. I have known people who have experienced precisely that type of healing. And yet, biblically, is that the promise for all believers at all times? Or, understanding laws and principles for biblical stewardship, do we have a part in how our own health experience plays out? As a principle of natural health and healing, understand that the best way to get rid of your disease, issue, problem, or condition is NOT to try and manage your complaints. The best way to free yourself of such bondage is to focus on spending more time, energy, effort, and resources actually "CREATING" the health you so desire. After all, most of us know or have experienced that it is possible to "manage" your signs and symptoms (discomfort) without ever realizing or creating any beneficial, long-term health or freedom gains. There is a saying: "Caged birds dream of flying...free birds just fly." Isn't it time for you to be set free, to come out from behind your bondage—that closed and restrictive environment that sickness and disease has placed upon you, and fly? Just fly...happy, healthy, and free! With that in mind, we present to you this work: a health success story that can model a path toward health, freedom, and wellness. Joe Horn knows first-hand the pain, suffering, and weight of "being held in a cage." His efforts and personal health journey have shown him that there is a more excellent way…a way out! A path to freedom. Joe knows the value and necessity that we all can benefit from knowing: How to "correct and continue" as we journey towards something better. It's NOT too late! Despite years or decades of ignorance or rebellion with poor decisions and lifestyle habits…now is the time! You, also, can correct and continue…a little wisdom…a little understanding…a little knowledge…coupled with a dollop of personal responsibility and the God-given mantle of stewardship for the "living temple" that He has so graciously provided as a vehicle for you and the Holy Spirit to live in and to express and demonstrate "A Living Jesus to a dying world."

Blessings!

…And may the Father of Lights shine brightly and bless you in directing you with all of your health goals and desires.

Yours in Him and in health!

Ralph A. Umbriaco, DC, MsTOM, CNHP

About the Author: Dr. Ralph Umbriaco's passion as a healthcare professional is to empower patients with the knowledge and understanding necessary for them to experience their own healing miracle. Rather than "fighting" or "focusing" on this concept that is called disease, why not, instead, invest and redirect an effective portion of our time, energies and effort in CREATING so much "real health" that disease and discomfort can no longer have any power over you, your life, you family or your environment? Dr. Umbriaco is a state-licensed doctor of chiropractic medicine and holds a private practice in Newport Beach, California. He also holds a master's of science in traditional oriental medicine (MSTOM) and is a certified natural health professional (CNHP).

Notes

1. Grieve, Carol. "Leaky Gut: Is It Becoming an Epidemic?" *Food Integrity Now*, 27 May 2015, http://foodintegritynow.org/2015/05/27/leaky-gut-is-it-becoming-an-epidemic/. Accessed 3 Jan. 2018.

2. Ibid.

3. *The Matrix*. DVD. Directed by Andy Wachowski and Larry Wachowski, Warner Bros. USA, 1999.

4. Coleman, Marilyn., Ganong, Lawrence H., and Warzinik, Kelly. *Family Life in the 20th-Century America*. Greenwood Press, Westport Connecticut, 2007. P. 51.

5. Ibid., P. 52.

6. Talty, Alexandra. "New Study Finds Millennials Spend 44 Percent of Food Dollars On Eating Out." *Forbes*, 17 Oct. 2017, https://www.forbes.com/sites/alexandratalty/2016/10/17/millennials-spend-44-percent-of-food-dollars-on-eating-out-says-food-institute/#1b5a3e8a3ff6. Accessed 19 Dec. 2017.

7. Lamagna, Maria. "Why Millennials Don't Know How to Cook." *Market Watch*, 10 Sept. 2016, http://www.marketwatch.com/story/why-millennials-dont-know-how-to-cook-2016-08-10. Accessed 18 Dec. 2017.

8. "Cooking Survey Reveals That 28% Of Americans Can't Cook." *Huffington Post*, 9 Sept. 2011, https://www.huffingtonpost.com/2011/09/09/cooking-survey_n_955600.html. Accessed 18 Dec. 2017.

9. Lawson, Helen. "Only One in Six Mothers Cooks from Scratch Each Day Because They Lack Time and Confidence in the Kitchen." *Daily mail*, 8 Mar 2013, http://www.dailymail.co.uk/news/article-2290106/Only-mothers-cooks-scratch-day-lack-time-confidence-kitchen.html. Accessed 18 Dec. 2017.

10. Taylor, Delano. "The Psychology of Colors." *Daily Infographic*, 19 Sept. 2012, http://www.dailyinfographic.com/the-psychology-of-colors-infographic. Accessed 19 Dec. 2017.

11. Winston Cigarettes. "Flintstones Winston Cigarettes Commercial (Rare)" Created [1954.] YouTube Video, 1:20. Posted [19 June 2006.] https://www.youtube.com/watch?v=FqdTBDkUEEQ.

12. Chan, Margaret. "The Changed Face of the Tobacco Industry." *World Health Organization*, 20 Mar. 2012, http://www.who.int/dg/speeches/2012/tobacco_20120320/en/. Accessed 18 Dec. 2017.

13. Ibid.

14. Bovay, John. "FDA Refusals of Imported Food Products by Country and Category, 2005-2013." *United States Department of Agriculture*, https://www.ers.usda.gov/webdocs/publications/44066/57014_eib151.pdf?v=42457. Accessed 18 Dec. 2017.

15. Ibid.

16. Roseboro, Ken. "Arpad Pusztai and the Risks of Genetic Engineering." *Organic Consumers* Association, 1 June 2009, https://www.organicconsumers.org/news/arpad-pusztai-and-risks-genetic-engineering. Accessed 18 Dec. 2017.

17. Smith, Jeffrey. "Throwing Biotech Lies at Tomatoes—Part 1: killer Tomatoes." *Huffington Post*, 31 Dec. 2010, https://www.huffingtonpost.com/jeffrey-smith/throwing-biotech-lies-at_b_803139.html. Accessed 19 Dec. 2017.

18. Ibid.

19. Dash, Pramod. "Blood-brain Barrier Maintains the Constancy of the Brain's Internal Environment." *Neuroscience Online*, http://nba.uth.tmc.edu/neuroscience/s4/chapter11.html. Accessed 19 Dec. 2017.

20. Brown, Edward. "Psychoneuroimmunology and Chiropractic." *J. Vertebral Subluxation Res. – JVSR.Com,*30 Sept. 2005. http://www.mccoypress.net/annals/docs/2005-1147_brown.pdf. Accessed 18 Dec. 2017.

21. Lant, Karla. "Excitotoxins: The FDA-Approved Way to Damage Your Brain." *Honey* Colony, 22 June 2015, https://www.honeycolony.com/article/excitotoxins-fda-approved-damage-brain/. Accessed 18 Dec. 2017.

22. Ibid.

23. Ibid.

24. Gunnars, Kris. "Daily Intake of Sugar—How Much Sugar Should You Eat Per Day?" 27 May 2017, https://www.healthline.com/nutrition/how-much-sugar-per-day. Accessed 18 Dec. 2017.

25. Welch, Ashley. "Do You Know How Much Sugar Is in Your Starbucks Drink?" 19 Feb. 2016, https://www.cbsnews.com/news/do-you-know-how-much-sugar-is-in-your-starbucks-drink/. Accessed 18 Dec. 2017.

26. Eilperin, Juliet. "US Sugar Industry Targets New Study," *The Washington Post*, 25 Apr 2003, https://www.washingtonpost.com/archive/politics/2003/04/23/us-sugar-industry-targets-new-study/5fe410ab-9f87-4e10-afbe-91cb2f2e6d05/?utm_term=.c674ec4634a8. Last Accessed 3 Feb. 2018.

27. Dobbins, Chris. "Report Offers New Eating and Physical Activity Targets to Reduce Chronic Disease Risk." *The National Academies of Sciences Engineering Medicine*, 5 Sept. 2002, http://www8.nationalacademies.org/onpinews/newsitem.aspx?RecordID=10490. Accessed 18 Dec. 2017.

28. MacPherson, Kitta. "Sugar Can Be Addictive, Princeton Scientist Says." *Princeton University Online*, 10 Dec. 2008, https://www.princeton.edu/news/2008/12/10/sugar-can-be-addictive-princeton-scientist-says. Accessed 18 Dec. 2017.

29. Ibid.

30. Black, Rosemary. "Sugar as Addictive as Cocaine, Heroin: Studies Suggest." *NY Daily News*, 11 Dec. 2008, http://www.nydailynews.com/life-style/health/sugar-addictive-cocaine-heroin-studies-suggest-article-1.356819. Accessed 18 Dec. 2017.

31. Bennett, Connie. "The Rats Who Preferred Sugar Over Cocaine." *HuffPost*, 10 Sept. 2010, https://www.huffingtonpost.com/connie-bennett/the-rats-who-preferred-su_b_712254.html. Accessed 18 Dec. 2017.

32. Lustig, Robert, *Fed Up: It's Time to Get Real About Food*. DVD. Directed by Stephanie Soechtig. USA, 9 May 2014. Time Stamp 27:12.

33. Mercola, Joseph. "Guess Who Funds High Fructose Corn Syrup Studies?" *Mercola Online*, 21 Oct. 2008, https://articles.mercola.com/sites/articles/archive/2008/10/21/guess-who-funds-high-fructose-corn-syrup-studies.aspx. Accessed 18 Dec. 2017.

34. Ibid.

35. Benson, Jonathan. "Corn Refiners Association sued for falsely claiming that high fructose corn syrup is same as sugar." *Natural* News, 24 Dec. 2011, https://www.naturalnews.com/034477_Corn_Refiners_Association_ HFCS_sugar.html. Accessed 18 Dec. 2017.

36. "Partnership for a Healthier America Announces Food and Beverage manufacturer Steps to Fight Childhood Obesity." *A Healthier America*, 17 May 2010, https://www.ahealthieramerica.org/articles/partnership-for-a-healthier-america-announces-food-and-beverage-manufacturer-steps-to-fight-childhood-obesity-334. Accessed 18 Dec. 2017.

37. Neal, Todd. "Health Insurers Hedge Bets with Fast Food Stock." *ABC News*, 16 April 2016, http://abcnews.go.com/Health/w_DietAndFitness/health-insurance-companies-invest-billions-fast-food-stock/story?id=10392603. Accessed 19 Dec. 2017.

38. Wang, Y., Beydoun, MA., Caballero, B., Kumanyika, SK. "Will All Americans Become Overweight or Obese? Estimating the Progression and Cost of the US Obesity Epidemic." *PubMed US National Library of Medicine; National Institutes of Health*, 16 Oct. 2008, https://www.ncbi.nlm. nih.gov/pubmed/18719634. Accessed 19 Dec. 2017.

39. Lustig, Robert, *Fed Up: It's Time to Get Real about Food*. DVD. Directed by Stephanie Soechtig. USA, 9 May 2014. Time Stamp 1:21:00-1:23:00.

40. Karp, Harvey, *Fed Up: It's Time to Get Real About Food*. DVD. Directed by Stephanie Soechtig. USA, 9 May 2014. Time Stamp 1:21:00-1:23:00.p

41. Mercola, Joseph. "How to Wean Yourself Off Processed Foods in 7 Steps." *Mercola Online*, 1 July 2010, https://articles.mercola.com/sites/articles/ archive/2010/07/01/wean-yourself-off-processed-foods-in-7-steps.aspx. Accessed 18 Dec. 2017.

42. Urry, Amelia. "Our Crazy Farm Subsidies, Explained." *Grist*, 20 April 2015, http://grist.org/food/our-crazy-farm-subsidies-explained/. Accessed 18 Dec. 2017.

43. Hyman, Mark. "The Toxic Triad: How Big Food, Big Farming, and Big Pharma Spread Obesity, Diabetes, and Chronic Disease Across the Globe." *Dr. Hyman Online*, 2016, http://drhyman.com/blog/2010/10/22/the-toxic-

triad-how-big-food-big-farming-and-big-pharma-spread-obesity-diabetes-and-chronic-disease-across-the-globe/. Accessed 18 Dec. 2017.

44. Loudon, Manette. "The FDA Exposed: An Interview with Dr. David Graham, the Vioxx Whistleblower." *Natural* News, 30 Aug. 2005, https://www.naturalnews.com/011401_Dr_David_Graham_the_FDA.html. Accessed 18 Dec. 2017.

45. Ibid.

46. Olsen, Gwen. Confessions of an RX Drug Pusher: God's Call to Loving Arms. iUniverse, Lincoln, NE, 2005. page 114.

47. Ibid., page 114.

48. Ibid., page 115.

49. Brown, Kristen. "The FDA Is Cracking Down on Homeopathic Remedies." *Gizmodo*, 18 Dec 2017, https://gizmodo.com/the-fda-is-cracking-down-on-homeopathic-remedies-1821403162?IR=T. Accessed 19 Dec. 2017.

50. Ibid.

51. Gregory, Christian A. and Coleman-Jensen, Alisha. "Food Insecurity, Chronic Disease, and Health Among Working-Age Adults." *United States Department of Agriculture*, July 2017, https://www.ers.usda.gov/webdocs/publications/84467/err-235.pdf?v=42942. Accessed 18 Dec. 2017.

52. Ibid.

53. Tiehen, Laura., Newman, Constance., and Kirlin, John A. "The Food-Spending Patterns of Households Participating in the Supplemental Nutrition Assistance Program: Findings from USDA's FoodAPS." *United States Department of Agriculture*, Aug 2017, https://www.ers.usda.gov/webdocs/publications/84467/err-235.pdf?v=42942. Accessed 18 Dec. 2017.

54. Ibid.

55. Okrent, Abigail M. and Kumcu, Aylin. "U.S. Households' Demand for Convenience Foods." *United States Department of Agriculture*, July 2016, https://www.ers.usda.gov/webdocs/publications/80654/err-211.pdf?v=42668. Accessed 18 Dec. 2017.

56. "Child Obesity Grows Tenfold in 40 Years." *Newsmax*, 11 Oct. 2017, https://www.newsmax.com/t/newsmax/article/818995/177. Accessed 18 Dec. 2017.

57. Ibid.

58. Kamb, Steve. "Why Sugar Is the Worst Thing Ever For You. Seriously. Ever." *Nerd Fitness*, https://www.nerdfitness.com/blog/everything-you-need-to-know-about-sugar/. Accessed 19 Dec. 2017.

59. Ibid.

60. Lant, Karla. "Excitotoxins: The FDA-Approved Way to Damage Your Brain." *Honey* Colony, 22 June 2015, https://www.honeycolony.com/article/excitotoxins-fda-approved-damage-brain/. Accessed 18 Dec. 2017.

61. "Obesity a Factor in 4 in 10 Cancers: CDC." *Newsmax Health*, 10 Oct. 2017, https://www.newsmax.com/Health/Health-News/obesity-cancer-cdc/2017/10/10/id/818878/. Accessed 18 Dec. 2017.

62. Ibid.

63. Ruderman, N., Chisholm, D., Pi-Sunyer, X., and Schneider, S. "The Metabolically Obese, Normal-Weight Individual Revisited." *American Diabetes Association: Diabetes Journals Online*, May 1998, http://diabetes.diabetesjournals.org/content/47/5/699. Accessed 18 Dec. 2017.

64. Hyman, Mark. "Are You a Skinny Fat person? 10 Steps to Cure the Skinny Fat Syndrome." *Huffpost*, 26 Aug. 2012, https://www.huffingtonpost.com/dr-mark-hyman/skinny-fat_b_1799797.html. Accessed 18 Dec. 2017.

65. Ibid.

66. "Energy Drinks Cost New Father Part of His Skull, Wife Claims." *Fox News*, 13 Oct. 2017, http://www.foxnews.com/lifestyle/2017/10/13/energy-drinks-cost-new-father-part-his-skull-wife-claims.html. Accessed 19 Dec. 2017.

67. Lant, Karla. "Excitotoxins: The FDA-Approved Way to Damage Your Brain." *Honey* Colony, 22 June 2015, https://www.honeycolony.com/article/excitotoxins-fda-approved-damage-brain/. Accessed 18 Dec. 2017.

68. Armstrong, Elizabeth. "Debate Grows over Antidepressant Use among Preschoolers." *The Christian Science Monitor*, 8 April 2004, https://www.csmonitor.com/2004/0408/p01s03-ussc.html. Accessed 18 Dec. 2017.

69. Ibid.

70. Antonia, KJ. "Why We Should Fear Preschoolers on Prozac." *Slate Magazine Online*, 2 Sept. 2010. http://www.slate.com/blogs/xx_factor/2010/09/02/diagnosing_depression_in_preschoolers_may_mean_therapy_for_the_rich_and_more_drugs_for_the_poor.html. Accessed 18 Dec. 2017.

71. Ibid.

72. Brown, Edward. "Psychoneuroimmunology and Chiropractic." *J. Vertebral Subluxation Res. – JVSR.Com,* 30 Sept. 2005. http://www.mccoypress.net/annals/docs/2005-1147_brown.pdf. Accessed 18 Dec. 2017.

73. Knopf, Taylor. "CDC: 'Nearly 50% of U.S. Adults Will Develop at Least One Mental Illness'." *CNS News*, 13 June 2013, https://www.cnsnews.com/news/article/cdc-nearly-50-us-adults-will-develop-least-one-mental-illness. Accessed 19 Dec. 2017.

74. Olsen, Gwen. Confessions of an RX Drug Pusher: God's Call to Loving Arms. iUniverse, Lincoln, NE, 2005. page 118.

75. Cerundolo, Aida. "Have You Seen Junior's Psyche Profile?" *The Wall Street Journal Online*, 8 May 2017, https://www.wsj.com/articles/have-you-seen-juniors-psych-profile-1494286467. Accessed 18 Dec. 2017.

76. Ibid.

77. Orwell, George. *1984*. Harville Secker, London, 1949.

78. Nowak, Peter. "How McDonald's Has Shaped the Food Biz." *CBC News*, 14 May 2015, http://www.cbc.ca/news/business/how-mcdonald-s-has-shaped-the-food-biz-1.3074081. Accessed 19 Dec. 2017.

79. Barlett, Donald L. and Steele, James B. "Monsanto's Harvest of Fear." *Vanity Fair Online*, May 2008, https://www.vanityfair.com/news/2008/05/monsanto200805. Accessed 18 Dec. 2017.

80. Ibid.

81. Ibid.

82. Ibid.

83. Ibid.

84. Edwards, Scott. "How a Family was Crushed & Made Homeless by Tyson Foods." *Elephant Journal Online*, 2 Dec. 2012, https://www.elephantjournal.com/2012/12/how-a-family-was-crushed-and-made-homeless-by-tyson-foods-scott-edwards/. Accessed 19 Dec. 2017.

85. Ibid.

86. Fesperman, Dan. and Shatzkin, Kate. "Taking a Stand, Losing the Farm." *The Baltimore Sun Online*, http://www.baltimoresun.com/business/bal-pecking-order-day2a-story.html. Accessed 18 Dec. 2017.

87. Wilkinson, Juliet. "Are Hormones in Meat Affecting Humans?" *Livestrong*,

14 Aug. 2017, https://www.livestrong.com/article/464430-are-hormones-in-meat-affecting-humans/. Accessed 18 Dec. 2017.

88. Jeong, Sang-Hee., Kang, Daejin., Lim, Myung-Woon., Kang, Chang Soo., and Sung, Ha Jung. "Risk Assessment of Growth Hormones and Antimicrobial Residues in Meat." *US National Library of Medicine: National Institutes of Health: Toxicological Research*, 26 Dec. 2010, https://www.ncbi.nlm.nih.gov/pmc/articles/PMC3834504/. Accessed 18 Dec. 2017.

89. The American Society medical and editorial content team. "Recombinant Bovine Growth Hormone." *American Cancer Society*, Last Revised 10 Sept. 2014, https://www.cancer.org/cancer/cancer-causes/recombinant-bovine-growth-hormone.html. Accessed 19 Dec. 2017.

90. Ibid.

91. Ipatenco, Sara. "The Effects of Drinking Milk That Contains Growth Hormones." *Livestrong*, 3 Oct. 2017, https://www.livestrong.com/article/375661-the-effects-of-drinking-milk-that-contains-growth-hormones/. Accessed 19 Dec. 2017.

92. Wal-Mart. "Wal-Mart Offers Private Label Milk Produced without Artificial Growth Hormone." *Wal-Mart*, 21 March 2008, https://corporate.walmart.com/_news_/news-archive/2008/03/24/wal-mart-offers-private-label-milk-produced-without-artificial-growth-hormone. Accessed 19 Dec. 2017.

93. Jeong, Sang-Hee., Kang, Daejin., Lim, Myung-Woon., Kang, Chang Soo., and Sung, Ha Jung. "Risk Assessment of Growth Hormones and Antimicrobial Residues in Meat." *US National Library of Medicine: National Institutes of Health: Toxicological Research*, 26 Dec. 2010, https://www.ncbi.nlm.nih.gov/pmc/articles/PMC3834504/. Accessed 18 Dec. 2017.

94. Ibid.

95. Ibid.

96. Ibid.

97. "Massive Increase in Aantimicrobials Use in Animals to Lead to Widespread Drug Resistance in Humans." *Homeland Security Newswire*, 9 Oct. 2017, http://www.homelandsecuritynewswire.com/dr20171009-massive-increase-in-antimicrobials-use-in-animals-to-lead-to-widespread-drug-resistance-in-humans. Accessed 18 Dec. 2017.

98. "Keep Hormones and Antibiotics off the Menu." *The Healthy Child*, 1 Oct. 2013, http://www.healthychild.org/easy-steps/keep-hormones-and-antibiotics-off-the-menu/. Accessed 18 Dec. 2017.

99. "Nonprofits Sue Third-Largest Poultry Co. for False Advertising of Drug-Contaminated Chicken." *Organic Consumers Association*, 22 June 2017, https://www.organicconsumers.org/press/nonprofits-sue-third-largest-poultry-co-false-advertising-drug-contaminated-chicken. Accessed 18 Dec. 2017.

100. Ibid.

101. "Massive Increase in Antimicrobials Use in Animals to Lead to Widespread Drug Resistance in Humans." *Homeland Security Newswire*, 9 Oct. 2017, http://www.homelandsecuritynewswire.com/dr20171009-massive-increase-in-antimicrobials-use-in-animals-to-lead-to-widespread-drug-resistance-in-humans. Accessed 18 Dec. 2017.

102. Ibid.

103. Ted Talks. "Factory Farms, Antibiotics and Superbugs: Lance Price at TEDxManhattan." Published [March 11, 2014.] YouTube video, 13:04. Posted [March 11, 2014.] https://www.youtube.com/watch?v=ZwHapgrF99A.

104. Scheer, Roddy., and Moss, Doug. "Dirt Poor: Have Fruits and Vegetables Become Less Nutritious?" *Scientific American*, https://www.scientificamerican.com/article/soil-depletion-and-nutrition-loss/. Accessed 18 Dec. 2017.

105. Davis, Donald R., Epp, Melvin D., and Riordan, Hugh D. "Changes in USDA Food Composition Data for 43 Garden Crops, 1950 to 1999." *Bio-Communications Research Institute, Wichita, Kansas. Biochemical Institute, The University of Texas, Austin, Texas.* http://citeseerx.ist.psu.edu/viewdoc/download?doi=10.1.1.611.9774&rep=rep1&type=pdf. Accessed 18 Dec. 2017.

106. Scheer, Roddy., and Moss, Doug. "Dirt Poor: Have Fruits and Vegetables Become Less Nutritious?" *Scientific American*, https://www.scientificamerican.com/article/soil-depletion-and-nutrition-loss/. Accessed 18 Dec. 2017.

107. Torres, Marco. "Soil Depletion and the Decline in Nutritional Content of Fruits and Vegetables." *Signs of the Times*, 3 Jan. 2017, https://www.sott. net/article/338538-Soil-depletion-and-the-decline-in-nutritional-content-of-fruits-and-vegetables. Accessed 18 Dec. 2017.

108. Robinson, Jo. "Breeding the Nutrition Out of Our Food." *The New York Times*, 25 May 2013, http://www.nytimes.com/2013/05/26/opinion/ sunday/breeding-the-nutrition-out-of-our-food.html?pagewanted=all. Accessed 18 Dec. 2017.

109. Paul, Katherine. "Monsanto Isn't Feeding the World—It's Killing Our Children." *Organic Consumers Association*, 9 March 2017, https://www. organicconsumers.org/blog/monsanto-isn%E2%80%99t-feeding-world%E2%80%94it%E2%80%99s-killing-our-children. Accessed 18 Dec. 2017.

110. Ibid.

111. Ibid.

112. Fano, Alix, *Lethal Laws*, 1997 page 108.

113. "Pollution (Water, Air, Chemicals)." *Food Empowerment Project* http:// www.foodispower.org/pollution-water-air-chemicals/. Accessed 18 Dec. 2017.

114. Ibid.

115. Donsky, Andrea. "7 Scary Food Additives to Avoid." *Naturally Savvy*, 1 Oct. 2013, http://naturallysavvy.com/eat/7-scary-food-additives-to-avoid. Accessed 6 Feb. 2018.

116. Mercola, Joseph. "7 Worst Ingredients in Food." *Mercola Online*, 30 Dec. 2013. https://articles.mercola.com/sites/articles/archive/2013/12/30/worst-food-ingredients.aspx. Accessed 6 Feb. 2018.

117. Goldschmidt, Vivian. "12 Dangerous and Hidden Food Ingredients in Seemingly Healthy Foods." *Save Our Bones Online*, https://saveourbones. com/12-dangerous-ingredients/, Accessed 6 Feb. 2018.

118. Perry, Cat. "The 9 Scariest Food Additives You're Eating Right Now." *Men's Fitness Online*, 8 Oct. 2016, https://www.mensfitness.com/nutrition/what-to-eat/9-scariest-food-additives-youre-eating-right-now. Accessed 6 Feb. 2018.

119. Blaylock, Russell. L. *Excitotoxins: The Taste That Kills*. New Mexico, Health Press, 1996.

120. Mercola, Joseph. "7 Worst Ingredients in Food." *Mercola Online*, 30 Dec. 2013. https://articles.mercola.com/sites/articles/archive/2013/12/30/worst-food-ingredients.aspx. Accessed 18 Dec. 2017.

121. Ibid.

122. Brown, Edward. "Psychoneuroimmunology and Chiropractic." *J. Vertebral Subluxation Res. – JVSR.Com,*30 Sept. 2005. http://www.mccoypress.net/annals/docs/2005-1147_brown.pdf. Accessed 18 Dec. 2017.

123. Mercola, Joseph. "7 Worst Ingredients in Food." *Mercola Online*, 30 Dec. 2013. https://articles.mercola.com/sites/articles/archive/2013/12/30/worst-food-ingredients.aspx. Accessed 18 Dec. 2017.

124. Cronin, Jeff. "In Europe, Dyed Foods Get Warning Label." *Center for Science in The Public Interest*, 20 July 2010, https://cspinet.org/new/201007201.html. Accessed 18 Dec. 2017.

125. Mercola, Joseph. "7 Worst ingredients in Food." *Mercola Online*, 30 Dec. 2013. https://articles.mercola.com/sites/articles/archive/2013/12/30/worst-food-ingredients.aspx. Accessed 18 Dec. 2017.

126. Donsky, Andrea. "7 Scary Food Additives to Avoid." *Naturally Savvy*, 1 Oct. 2013, http://naturallysavvy.com/eat/7-scary-food-additives-to-avoid. Accessed 18 Dec. 2017.

127. Ibid

128. Mercola, Joseph. "7 Worst Ingredients in Food." *Mercola Online*, 30 Dec. 2013. https://articles.mercola.com/sites/articles/archive/2013/12/30/worst-food-ingredients.aspx. Accessed 18 Dec. 2017.

129. Perry, Cat. "The 9 Scariest Food Additives You're Eating Right Now." *Men's Fitness Online*, 8 Oct. 2016, https://www.mensfitness.com/nutrition/what-to-eat/9-scariest-food-additives-youre-eating-right-now. Accessed 18 Dec. 2017.

130. Brownstein, David. *Heal Your Leaky Gut: The Hidden Cause of Many Chronic Diseases*. Humanix Books, Palm Beach, FL. 2017.

131. "Blood Test: Immunoglobulins (IgA, IgG, IgM)." *Kid's Health* http://kidshealth.org/en/parents/test-immunoglobulins.html. Accessed 18 Dec. 2017.

132. https://www.usatoday.com/story/money/business/2017/12/05/nestle-buy-health-products-maker-atrium-2-3-billion/923679001/

133. Brownstein, David. *Heal Your Leaky Gut: The Hidden Cause of Many Chronic Diseases*. Humanix Books, Palm Beach, FL. 2017. Page 139.

134. Group, Edward. "3 Reasons Healthy Gut Flora Is Important." *Global Healing Center*, 19 April 2015, https://www.globalhealingcenter.com/ natural-health/3-reasons-healthy-gut-flora-are-important/. Accessed 18 Dec. 2017.

135. Robertson, Ruairi. "Why the Gut Microbiome Is Crucial for Your Health." *Healthline: Authority Nutrition*, 27 June 2017, https://www.healthline.com/ nutrition/gut-microbiome-and-health. Accessed 18 Dec. 2017.

136. Ibid.

137. Ibid.

138. Ibid.

139. "Good Gut Bugs Help Cancer Immunotherapy Drugs Work." *Newsmax*, 3 Nov. 2017, https://www.newsmax.com/health/health-news/microbiome-gut-microbes-immunotherapy/2017/11/03/id/823902/. Accessed 18 Dec. 2017.

140. Robertson, Ruairi. "Why the Gut Microbiome Is Crucial for Your Health." *Healthline: Authority Nutrition*, 27 June 2017, https://www.healthline.com/ nutrition/gut-microbiome-and-health. Accessed 18 Dec. 2017.

141. Lord, Douglas. "Your Body's Second Brain—The Importance of Gut Health." *Nava Health & Vitality Center*, 1 June 2015, http://www. navacenter.com/community/article-library/browse/2015/06/01/your-body's-second-brain---the-importance-of-gut-health. Accessed 18 Dec. 2017.

142. Pomeroy, Ross. "Alzheimer's Patients Have Altered Gut Bacteria." *RealClear Science*, 23 Oct. 2017, https://www.realclearscience.com/quick_and_clear_ science/2017/10/23/alzheimers_patients_have_altered_gut_bacteria.html. Accessed 18 Dec. 2017.

143. Ibid.

144. Brownstein, David. *Heal Your Leaky Gut: The Hidden Cause of Many Chronic Diseases*. Humanix Books, Palm Beach, FL. 2017. Page 68–69.

145. Rossi, Carey. "11 Reasons Why You're Not Losing Belly Fat." *Health*, 1 Nov. 2016, http://www.health.com/health/gallery/0,,20807507,00. html#you-re-skimping-on-sleep-0. Accessed 18 Dec. 2017.

146. Weil, Andrew and Becker, Brian. "Finding Good Vitamins." *Andrew Weil Online*, Updated on 24 Feb. 2014, https://www.drweil.com/vitamins-supplements-herbs/vitamins/finding-good-vitamins/. Accessed 18 Dec. 2017.

147. Mercola, Joseph. "How to Wean Yourself Off Processed Foods in 7 Steps." *Mercola Online*, 1 July 2010, https://articles.mercola.com/sites/articles/archive/2010/07/01/wean-yourself-off-processed-foods-in-7-steps.aspx. Accessed 18 Dec. 2017.

148. Hinckley, David. "Average American Watches 5 Hours of TV per Day, Report Shows." *NY Daily News*, 5 March 2014, http://www.nydailynews.com/life-style/average-american-watches-5-hours-tv-day-article-1.1711954. Accessed 18 Dec. 2017.

149. Best, Shivali. "Is THIS Why Your Mum's Meals Taste So Good? Food 'Made with Love' Really Is More Delicious, Claims Study." *Daily Mail: Science & Tech*, 5 Dec. 2016, http://www.dailymail.co.uk/sciencetech/article-4001694/Is-mum-s-meals-taste-good-Food-love-really-delicious-claims-study.html. Accessed 18 Dec. 2017.

150. Brownstein, David. *Heal Your Leaky Gut: The Hidden Cause of Many Chronic Diseases*. Humanix Books, Palm Beach, FL. 2017. Page 25.

151. Blonz, Edward R. "How to Buy Produce." *Berkeley Wellness*, 15 Aug. 2013, http://www.berkeleywellness.com/healthy-eating/food/article/how-buy-produce. Accessed 18 Dec. 2017.

152. Mercola, Joseph. "How to Wean Yourself Off Processed Foods in 7 Steps." *Mercola Online*, 1 July 2010, https://articles.mercola.com/sites/articles/archive/2010/07/01/wean-yourself-off-processed-foods-in-7-steps.aspx. Accessed 18 Dec. 2017.

153. Ibid.

154. "'If You Can't Pronounce It, Don't Eat It'…Commonly Seen Quote." *Metabunk*, https://www.metabunk.org/if-you-cant-pronounce-it-dont-eat-it-commonly-seen-quote.t4751/. Accessed 18 Dec. 2017.

155. Hyman, Mark. "Are You a Skinny Fat Person? 10 Steps to Cure the Skinny Fat Syndrome." *Dr. Hyman Online*, 26 Aug. 2012, http://drhyman.com/blog/2012/08/17/are-you-a-skinny-fat-person-10-steps-to-cure-the-skinny-fat-syndrome/. Accessed 18 Dec. 2017.

156. Mercola, Joseph. "7 Worst Ingredients in Food." *Mercola Online*, 30 Dec. 2013. https://articles.mercola.com/sites/articles/archive/2013/12/30/worst-food-ingredients.aspx. Accessed 18 Dec. 2017.

157. "Understanding Food Labels: The many labels on our food, from organic vegetables to USDA-inspected meat to cage-free eggs, can be confusing. How much do food labels actually tell you?" *Food & Water Watch*, https://www.foodandwaterwatch.org/about/live-healthy/consumer-labels. Accessed 18 Dec. 2017.

158. Barone, Jeanine. "Can You Trust Calorie Counts?" *Berkeley Wellness*, 30 Sept. 2016, http://www.berkeleywellness.com/healthy-eating/nutrition/article/can-you-trust-calorie-counts. Accessed 18 Dec. 2017.

159. Ibid.

160. Devries, Stephen. "5 Misleading Food Labels." *Gaples Institute for Integrative Cardiology*, https://www.gaplesinstitute.org/5-misleading-food-labels/. Accessed 18 Dec. 2017.

161. "Understanding Food Labels: The many labels on our food, from organic vegetables to USDA-inspected meat to cage-free eggs, can be confusing. How much do food labels actually tell you?" *Food & Water Watch*, https://www.foodandwaterwatch.org/about/live-healthy/consumer-labels. Accessed 18 Dec. 2017.

162. Ibid.

163. Ibid.

164. Ibid.

165. Clare, Mary. "USDA to Propose Standards for Organic Seafood Raised in U.S." 16 April, 2015, https://www.pbs.org/newshour/politics/usda-propose-standards-organic-seafood-raised-u-s. Accessed 19 Dec. 2017.

166. "Understanding Food Labels: The many labels on our food, from organic vegetables to USDA-inspected meat to cage-free eggs, can be confusing. How much do food labels actually tell you?" *Food & Water Watch*, https://www.foodandwaterwatch.org/about/live-healthy/consumer-labels. Accessed 18 Dec. 2017.

167. Kamb, Steve. "How to Not Get Scammed by Food Labels." *Nerd Fitness*, https://www.nerdfitness.com/blog/how-to-not-get-scammed-by-food-labels-plus-were-hiring/. Accessed 18 Dec. 2017.

168. Ibid.

169. Ibid.

170. Devries, Stephen. "5 Misleading Food Labels." *Gaples Institute for Integrative Cardiology*, https://www.gaplesinstitute.org/5-misleading-food-labels/. Accessed 18 Dec. 2017.

171. Ibid.

172. Kamb, Steve. "How to Not Get Scammed by Food Labels." *Nerd Fitness*, https://www.nerdfitness.com/blog/how-to-not-get-scammed-by-food-labels-plus-were-hiring/. Accessed 18 Dec. 2017.

173. Ibid.

174. "Understanding Food Labels: The many labels on our food, from organic vegetables to USDA-inspected meat to cage-free eggs, can be confusing. How much do food labels actually tell you?" *Food & Water Watch*, https://www.foodandwaterwatch.org/about/live-healthy/consumer-labels. Accessed 18 Dec. 2017.

175. Ibid.

176. Ibid.

177. Dewey, Caitlin. "A Growing Number of Young Americans Are Leaving Desk Jobs to Farm." *The Washington Post*, 23 Nov. 2017, https://www.washingtonpost.com/business/economy/a-growing-number-of-young-americans-are-leaving-desk-jobs-to-farm/2017/11/23/e3c018ac-c64c-11e7-afe9-4f60b5a6c4a0_story.html?utm_term=.4892b861ed7a. Accessed 18 Dec. 2017.

178. Ibid.

179. Ibid.

180. Hari, Vani. "How to Eat Organic on aBudget (Over 75 Tips!)." *Food Babe Online*, https://foodbabe.com/2013/05/20/how-to-eat-organic-on-a-budget/. Accessed 18 Dec. 2017.

181. Whitney, Donald S. *Spiritual Disciplines for the Christian Life*. Tyndale House Publishers, Colorado Springs, CO, 1991, 2014. Page 192.

182. Whitney, Donald S. *Spiritual Disciplines for the Christian Life*. Tyndale House Publishers, Colorado Springs, CO, 1991, 2014. Page 199.

183. Arthur Wallis, *God's Chosen Fast*. Christian Literature Crusade, Fort Washington, PA, 1968. Page 42.

184. Mathews, Jessica. "Fasting: A Trending Food Idea and New Frontier in Longevity Science." *CNBC Online: Modern Medicine*, 20 Oct. 2017, https://www.cnbc.com/2017/10/20/science-diet-fasting-may-be-more-important-than-just-eating-less.html. Accessed 18 Dec. 2017.

185. Ibid.

186. http://cim.med.miami.edu/clinical-services/acupuncture/ common-conditions-treated-acupuncture.

187. Bhatia, Manish. "What Is Homeopathy? Definition and Details." *Hpathy*.com, Nov. 2009. https://hpathy.com/abc-homeopathy/what-is-homeopathy-definition-and-details/. Accessed 6 Feb. 2018.

188. Bhatia, Manish. "Homeopathic FAQ." *Hpathy.com*. Oct. 2009. https:// hpathy.com/abc-homeopathy/homeopathic-faq. Accessed 6 Feb. 2018.